AF411934

THE HEADACHE BOOK

Edda Hanington, MD, MRCP

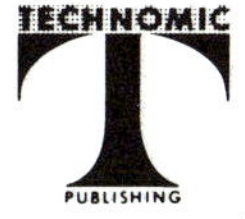

a **TECHNOMIC**® publication
TECHNOMIC Publishing Co., Inc.
265 Post Road West, Westport, CT. 06880

THE HEADACHE BOOK

by Edda Hanington

a **TECHNOMIC**[H] publication

Printed in U.S.A.
Library of Congress Card No. 80-52621
ISBN-87762-292-2

This book is dedicated to
my very dear husband John

"Let nothing disturb you,
Nothing alarm you.
All things are passing
God never changes . . ."

St. Teresa of Avila,
1515-1582
Patron Saint of Headache Sufferers.

The following pictures are included in this book by courtesy of The Wellcome Trustees.

The Headache by George Cruikshank, 1835.
The Four Humors from C. Ripa, Iconologia. Padua P.P. Tozzi, 1610/1611.
The Circle of Willis. Engraving of a drawing by Sir Christopher Wren from T. Willis *Cerebri anatome.* London; J. Flesher, 1664, Fig. 1.
The Cholic Engraving by George Cruikshank, 1835.
Hippocrates Engraving by Mecon after a drawing by Vauthier of a marble bust in the Louvre.
Galen (c. 129-200 A.D.) Engraving by G.P. Busch
Trephined Skull from New Britain In the Wellcome Museum, London.
Trephining; use of cranial elevator. From H. Brunschwig, "The noble experyence of the vertuous handyworks of surgeri". London, 1525.
Engraving Melencolia by Albrecht Durer from Friedrich Nuchter "Albrecht Durer", Ansbach, 1911.
The Nightmare Lithograph by M.Z.D. Schmidt, c.1800.
Chinese Acupuncture Chart In the Wellcome Institute Nicholas Culpeper (1616-1654) Engraving by Cross, 1650.
Queen Victoria (1819-1901) Engraving by D.J. Pound
Victoria Adelaide Mary Louise (1840-1901) Princess Royal and German Empress.

From Vienna Oesterreichische Nationalbibliothek MS 93, fol. 19 R. Test. "Plantain root, hung round the neck, takes away pain of the head marvellously".
13th century.

The picture illustrating Tension Headache is included by courtesy of Arbeitsmiljo, Stockholm, Sweden.

CONTENTS

INTRODUCTION

The pattern of human disease changes constantly. Improved living conditions, the introduction of new drugs and increasing knowledge about the causes of disease all contribute to this change. For example, smallpox has only come under control and been virtually eradicated in the last few years. In the western world tuberculosis and rheumatic fever are no longer rampant as they were even 30 years ago. Headaches, however, have always been with us and I doubt very much whether their incidence has altered greatly with time. Headaches are recorded in the earliest writings known to man. Five thousand years ago the Sumerians of Mesopotamia founded the world's first known civilization. They had a great deal in common with us today for they lived in cities, studied the stars, used a wheel and compiled a legal code. Since they built with mud bricks, however, and not in stone, it was only in the middle of the 19th Century that archeologists began to explore the shapeless mounds which concealed the secrets of their past. Writing began when the Sumarians wanted to label their stores and started marking small tags with drawings. They made engravings with a sharply pointed reed stylus on damp clay, and the tags were used to identify the stores. These marks were wedge shaped but gradually more complex symbols evolved and writing had begun.

Whenever things go wrong we tend to look for something or somebody to blame. So we can hardly be surprised when we find that in olden days disease was believed to be due to the gods. Evil spirits were considered responsible for pain and our forefathers went to alarming lengths in their attempts to drive these evil spirits away. For example, they made holes in the skull of the person afflicted with severe headaches in order to allow the evil spirits to escape. Many of these trephined skulls, dating back to the Bronze and Iron ages, have been found in the last 100 years. The belief that human ills are due to evil spirits is still held by the most primitive men alive today. They are the aborigines of Central Australia, where the medicine man still applies suction to the affected area of the patient in order to extract the spirit responsible for the symptoms.

Medical treatment remained in the province of religion or magic until about 500 years before the birth of Christ when Hippocrates was born on the Island of Cos, close to the coast of Asia minor. Hippocrates was the father of medicine and introduced reason and order into the way that human disease was regarded.

Despite the fact that Hippocrates knew little anatomy or physiology and had none of the basic tools of clinical medicine such as a thermometer or stethoscope, he taught with sound common sense. He made little use of the drugs of his day and relied upon nature as the greatest healer. He considered that climate played a major role in influencing the mind and body and refuted the idea that disease was a punishment inflicted by the gods. Hippocrates believed that "Every disease has its own nature and arises from external causes, from cold, from the sun or from changing winds". It was the Hippocratic School that introduced the humoral concept. This concept held sway for over 1000 years, and was accepted by Aristotle and strengthened in the 2nd Century A.D. by Galen.

Basically the humoral concept put forward the view that

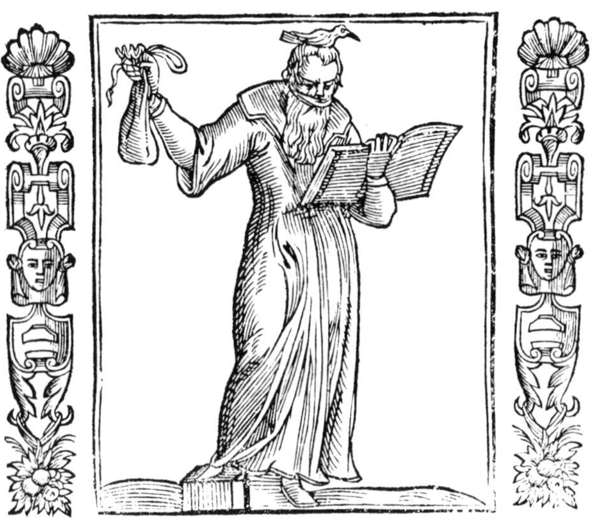

Figure 1. Malenconico per la Terra.

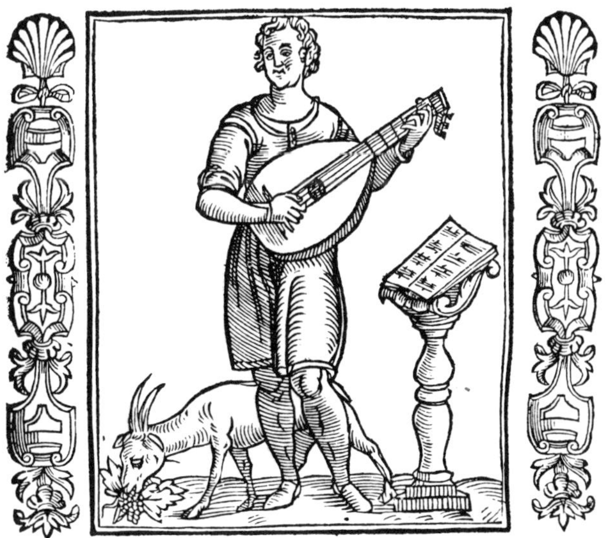

Figure 2. Sangvigno per L'Aria.

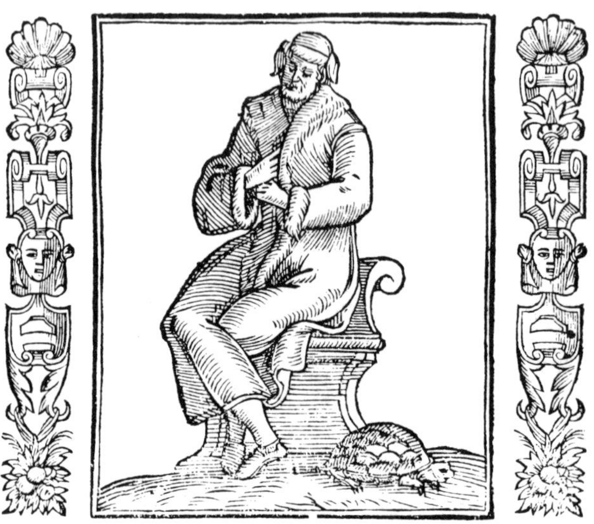

Figure 3. Flemmatico per L'Acqva.

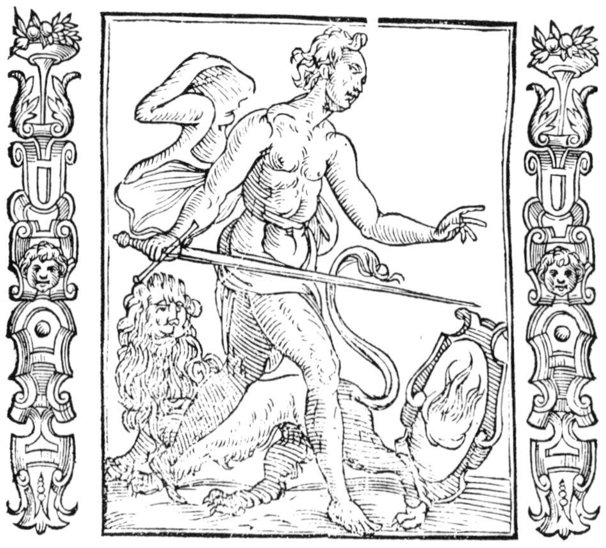

Figure 4. Colerico per Il Fvoco.

the human body contains 4 humors or fluids and that disease results when the balance of these humors is disturbed. The 4 humors were black bile, yellow bile, phlegm and blood. These 4 humors were thought to be associated not only with bodily disease but also with temperament. Thus black bile was associated with the choleric or easily roused to anger temperament. The other three temperaments were the melancholic, phlegmatic and sanguine. Human nature does not change and while the humoral theory of disease has long since ceased to be current the four temperaments are as recognizable now as they were when the humoral concept was firmly held.

Because of the major role which an excess of body fluids or plethora played in ancient pathology it is not surprising that headache was often attributed to an excess of fluid in the head. Hebrew teachings in the first centuries after Christ are recorded in the Talmud, and here we read that a special feature of generalized plethora is "the blood of the head". We also learn in these writings that a headache can be healed by rubbing the head with wine, vinegar or oil. Another suggestion is that the blood of a freshly slaughtered cock should be dripped over the painful area of the head. The carcass should then be hung at the sufferer's door so that he or she could rub the affected area of the head against it when going in or out of the dwelling.

One would imagine that the headache sufferer would need to feel fairly desperate before complying with these repellent instructions. In contrast, the Talmud also contains the more attractive advice that a white rose on a single stem should be boiled in water and the rose water applied to the aching head. And now, having recognised that there is nothing new under the sun as far as headaches are concerned, we can move on to consider the common causes of pain in the head.

CLASSIFICATION OF HEADACHE

"Common things commonly occur"

In 1962 an ad hoc Committee consisting of five physicians who were all experts on the subject of headache met to consider the classification of headache. They subsequently compiled a report which was published in the Journal of the American Medical Association[1].

In this report headaches were divided into 15 different categories. the first group was: *Vascular headaches of migraine type.*

Vascular headaches are those in which changes occur in the size and tone of blood vessels. Vascular headaches have certain characteristic features. The pain of vascular headaches is easily recognizable. It throbs with every heart beat and is made worse by any physical effort. Such acts as lifting up a suitcase or bending down to pick up an object from the floor, or even coughing, greatly increase the pain. The vascular group of headaches includes migraine. There are a number of types of migraine including such variants as cluster headache.

---

[1]Journal of American Medical Association, 1962, *179*, 717-718.

The second large category of headache listed by the Committee was: *Muscular contraction headache.*

This is by far the commonest type of headache encountered in clinical practice. It is often called "tension headache" and will only be mentioned here in passing, as there is a whole chapter in this book on the subject of tension headache. Occasionally vascular headache and muscle contraction headache occur together in the same patient. Patients with both types of headache suffer from headaches which resemble migraine in some respects but which differ from migraine because the pain is almost continuously present.

The Committee listed another separate category of *Non-Migrainous Vascular Headaches.*

Patients with a raised blood pressure sometimes complain of headache. This type of headache is included in this category. The headache is most often felt across the back of the head when the sufferer first wakes in the morning and usually wears off gradually when he (or she) gets up and begins his daily activities.

Climbers at high altitudes sometimes develop headaches which are due to vascular changes. The headaches occurring with acute infections, such as influenza, also fall into this category, as does the headache of a hangover. In a similar way to alcohol, some drugs can cause vascular headaches. For example, patients with anginal chest pain sometimes complain of a thumping headache when they take trinitrin tablets to relieve their chest pain. Trinitrin dilates the blood vessels in the body, thus relieving the pain caused by the constriction of vessels supplying the heart muscle, but in some patients this dilation also produces flushing of the face and headache symptoms.

The Committee which classified headaches listed a stress reaction headache in which pain is felt around the nose and the nose feels blocked. These nasal symptoms are not due to any allergy or infection but seem to result from the way in which some people react to stress.

Diseases of the eyes, ears or teeth can be responsible for less common causes of headache.

Infection in any part of the head can cause pain. This category includes infection within the skull, such as meningitis but this is obviously rare. Headache can also follow traumatic injury to the head and neck.

Depressed people sometimes complain of constant headaches. They often wake early in the morning, usually between 4:00 a.m. and 6:00 a.m., and cannot get off to sleep again.

There are some extremely rare causes of headache. These include the neuralgias which affect individual cranial nerves arising from the brain. Trigeminal neuralgia affects the fifth cranial nerve and is dealt with in a separate chapter in this book. This condition is sometimes confused with cluster headache to which another chapter is devoted.

The possibility of a brain tumor is the fear that haunts many headache sufferers. Anyone who reads the chapter in this book on tension headache and migraine will readily realize how the worry resulting from this fear will aggravate the headache symptoms already present and thus increase the anxiety. A vicious cycle of anxiety and headache is created which could have been avoided had the sufferer obtained medical advice at an earlier stage. Brain tumors are extremely rare. Tension headache is extremely common, and in the practice of medicine one must always remember that common things commonly occur.

INVESTIGATING HEADACHE

If you consult your doctor because you are suffering from headaches he will probably make a diagnosis on the basis of what you tell him combined with a clinical examination. However, your doctor may consider that some further investigations are needed and starting with the common investigations and moving to the rare, these are likely to be among the following:

Blood Count

Blood is composed of red cells, white cells and plasma. The red cells are made in bone marrow and are red because of their haemoglobin content. Haemoglobin is an iron containing pigment which carries oxygen from the lungs to all the cells of the body. The normal red cell count is around 5.0 million per cu.mm. of blood. It is slightly less in women and more in men. The normal haemoglobin level, which reflects the iron content and oxygen carrying capacity of the blood is 13 to 16 g/100 ml. When a complete blood count is done the size, shape and volume of the red cells is measured and reveals whether or not anaemia is a possible contributory factor to the symptoms from which a patient is suffering.

The white cells are also counted and inspected. The

normal white cell count is approximately 6000 to 10,000 per 1cu.mm of blood. There are a number of different types of white cells. Although some are made in the bone marrow, most of them are formed in the lymph nodes, thymus and spleen.

The total number of white cells usually increases in the presence of an acute bacterial infection whereas it may remain normal or fall with a viral infection. A detailed study of the blood is important in a wide variety of illnesses. In glandular fever, for example, the total white cell count may fall but the proportion of one type of white cell to another changes, and a certain type of white cell, called a monocyte, increases in number.

Sedimentation Rate

The E.S.R. or erythrocyte sedimentation rate is often done. The erythrocytes are red blood cells and this test estimates the rate at which they settle to the bottom of a narrow glass tube. The rate is increased in some forms of anemia and in a number of acute conditions such as rheumatoid arthritis. It is also markedly raised in one particular type of headache, called temporal arteritis. This occurs most frequently in people between the ages of fifty and eighty and the pain affects the temporal arteries which can be felt beating just in front of the ears. A raised E.S.R. is an indication that some associated condition should be sought with the diagnosis of headache.

Urine Examination

The examination of a specimen of urine is a routine part of a clinical check. It may reveal such conditions as diabetes, if sugar is detected, or possibly kidney trouble if protein is found.

Electroencephalogram (E.E.G.)

In this investigation small electrodes are placed at various points on the skull and the tiny electrical waves which they pick up from the activity at the surface of the brain are recorded. This is a painless, harmless, inexpensive test which sometimes produces helpful information. It is described in greater detail in the section on migraine and epilepsy.

X-Rays

Skull and chest X-rays are sometimes included in the investigation of patients with headaches.

Brain Scan

X-rays were discovered in 1895 and within a year had found a use in diagnostic medicine. One of the greatest technical advances in investigative medicine in the late twentieth century has been the advent of brain scanning techniques. These have superseded the rather unpleasant methods which had to be used previously in attempts to determine what was going on inside the skull. Brain scanning techniques are based on the fact that radionuclide materials, such as technetium 99m ($^{99}Tc^m$) are taken up in greater concentration by fluid spaces or blood in brain tissue and when serial pictures are taken over a period of 1 to 4 hours by an appropriate gamma camera any deviation from the normal presentation can be detected on the scan. Density differences as small as 0.5% can be picked out in the tissues. This highly sophisticated technique is nevertheless so simple that it can be used on an outpatient basis and causes the patient no discomfort.

TENSION HEADACHE

And when I found the door was locked,
I pushed and pulled and kicked and knocked.
                    Lewis Carroll, 1887.

The term "Stress Disorders" has been used to describe some of the illnesses that afflict modern man. Thus conditions like coronary heart disease and gastric ulcers are placed in this category as well as a large number of less dramatic chronic disorders such as certain skin diseases. Whether or not the stresses and strains to which man is subject today are any greater than those which affected his primordial ancestors is a debatable point. The necessity to hunt for food and clothing in the jungle in order to survive must have presented formidable problems but possibly part of the answer lies in the fact that our reactions to situations are largely conditioned by the age and society in which we live.

Be that as it may, tension headache is the headache most commonly encountered in clinical practice. In a headache survey conducted in a busy neurological out-patient clinic, nearly 70% of the headache sufferers were found to have tension headache. Tension headache can arise for the first time at any age from childhood onwards and is roughly twice as common in women as in men.

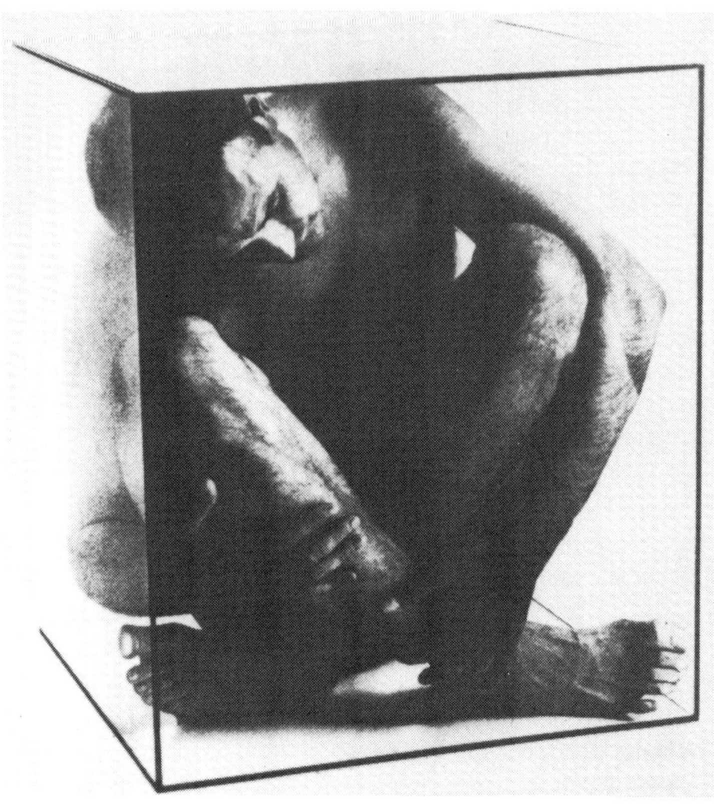

We have only to think of our physical state when we are held up in a traffic jam, while in a hurry to reach our destination, to realize that mental tension causes a tightening in muscles. In chronic tension headache pain is felt in the muscles of the head and neck which become taut and sometimes tender to touch. Occasionally the pain is felt on one side of the head only but it may spread to the muscles of the temples and forehead or be limited to these areas. Patients with tension headache often complain of a muzzy feeling. The pain is a dull, persistent ache which may be present for days or months or even years. It is often described as feeling like a weight on top of the head or like a gripping vice or tight band around the head like a skull cap. The pain of tension headache frequently gets worse during the afternoon and evening of the day and it is often relieved by rest or a change of scene. Not surprisingly the sufferer from tension headache may feel tired and exhausted and not infrequently depressed. Early morning waking with the inability to return to sleep is typical of this depression, and these chronic worriers might do well to reflect on Emerson's translation of an old French proverb:

"Some of your griefs you have cured
and the sharpest you still have survived
But what torments of pain you endured
From evils that never arrived."

Roughly one in every ten tension headache sufferers also suffer from migraine. These are the patients who, while describing typical attacks of migraine, state that they are never free of headache.

On rare occasions an attack of acute tension headache can arise with a dramatic onset. The sufferer complains of a sudden, severe pain in the head which may feel as if it is bursting. Blurring of vision and vomiting may add to the symptoms and a doctor is likely to be called. He will need to make a careful clinical examination to exclude much rarer causes of acute headache but the patient invariably recovers with rest and analgesic therapy.

There may be difficulty in distinguishing between migraine and tension headache and this difficulty is illustrated by the published correspondence between Queen Victoria and her eldest daughter "Vicky". The Princess Royal "Vicky" was born in 1840 and married the Crown Prince of Prussia at the age of 18. She became the mother of Emperor Wilhelm II who was the German Kaiser at the beginning of the first World War in 1914. Both Queen Victoria and her daughter suffered from recurrent severe headaches and provide a new interpretation of the proverb "Uneasy lies the head that wears the crown." In Cecil Woodham Smith's fascinating biography of the Queen frequent headache attacks were recorded. They invariably occurred in association with one of the numerous domestic or social upheavals with which the unenviable Queen's days were fraught. She could not have been other than acutely aware of the way in which frustration, disappointment and fatigue can precipitate headache attacks. At least the Queen must have found consolation in the fact that her daughter's own headaches gave her insight into her mother's problems. In a letter dated July 7th, 1868 the Crown Princess wrote in reply to a letter which she had received from her mother, in the following sympathetic and encouraging words:

"Many thanks for your dear letter received yesterday. Your description of what you feel is exactly how I felt in the month of March — the very rustling of a person's gown used to irritate me, and more than one person talking in the room made me feel as if I was going wild. I was ready to cry if I heard anyone speak for a few minutes together, and talking myself made a lump come in my throat! All this is so completely gone now that I have only the recollection left, but that is enough to make me sympathize with you. A complete change will I hope do you a great deal of good to diminish all these disagreeable and uncomfortable sensations — which must make you feel less up to anything. I believe nothing is better for the nerves than rising very early and having a walk before breakfast, and going early to rest — but this I think you do not like and it does not suit you. For me it does wonders."

As anticipated the advice proffered met with little enthusiasm, and the Queen replied in a letter written three days later:

"Going to bed early and getting up early would be a total impossibility for me. The night is the only quiet time for me — and I feel able to work then and not in the morning early."

Sufferers from tension headache often worry about the possibility that there is something seriously wrong with them. The worst fears are usually centered on the unspoken and often unspeakable possibility of a brain tumor or a stroke. Brain tumors and strokes are, of course, much more rare than tension headache is common. Since worry only adds to the symptoms already present, however, it is always wise to obtain medical advice and reassurance for any headache symptoms. The immediate effective treatment of tension headache is reassurance, possibly treatment with a mild tranquilizer for a short period of time and analgesic therapy. This is usually rapidly effective.

Chronic tension headache should not be a self-made diagnosis. It is a condition that can only be diagnosed after the patient has given the doctor a history and a careful clinical examination has been made. In particular the physician will wish to check the patient's blood pressure and it is only after he has found that all is in good order that he can explain the nature of tension headache. This explanation alone is often enough to relieve the worst symptoms. If the headaches persist the doctor may prescribe a mild tranquilizer to help relieve the tension and the analgesics commonly in use to help the pain. Drug treatment, however, can only allay the symptoms or camouflage the nature of tension headache. If we want to get to the root of any problem then we have to deal as far as we can with its cause. And this is where most headache sufferers need to pause for thought.

Things often are as bad as they seem and do not turn out "alright". However, we are forced to accept what we cannot alter and to push, pull, kick and knock when the door is firmly locked can only result in further tension and strain, and in so many cases, tension headaches. Perhaps this old prayer was particularly intended for just this group of headache sufferers.

> "God, grant me the serenity to accept the
> things I cannot change . . .
> Courage to change the things I can and
> wisdom to know the difference."

TEMPORAL ARTERITIS

In 1890 a physician called Hutchinson described a man who had "red streaks on his head".

The red streaks were his temporal arteries and they were red because they were inflamed and painful. If you place your fingers in front of your ears you can feel your temporal arteries beating. In temporal arteritis these arteries become thickened, tortuous and tender and the pulse can no longer be felt.

The condition of temporal arteritis, and the fact that it may occasionally be associated with a more general arterial disease in the body called polymyalgia rheumatica, was only clearly recognized in the latter half of last century. It is roughly as common as gout and is rare under the age of 50. It usually affects people over the age of 65 and the sufferers are invariably Caucasian. Both men and women can be afflicted. Pain is usually the first symptom that arises. It may occur in paroxysms and be felt initially in the jaw, scalp, tongue or neck, often on both sides of the head. Sometimes patients with temporal arteritis complain of neck stiffness but the symptoms in this disorder are characteristically vague. There is usually a sense of ill health, tiredness and loss of weight. The sufferer often becomes anaemic and runs a temperature in the evenings, and may have night sweats. In the rare instances where the more generalised disorder polymyalgia rheumatica develops then pain and stiffness start affecting the shoulder girdle and around the hips. This pain and stiffness has been known to be so sudden and so severe that the victim may wake one morning and be unable to get out of bed. He or she may then have to roll out of bed onto the floor in an attempt to get up, or call for assistance and be helped to rise. Another disorder in which morning stiffness is characteristic is rheumatoid arthritis, but in rheumatoid arthritis the pain and stiffness are felt chiefly in the small joints of the hands and feet whereas in polymyalgia rheumatica the stiffness and pain affect the trunk of the body and not the extremities.

Fortunately pain usually sends us scurrying to the doctor for help and it is particularly important in the case of temporal arteritis that help should be obtained as quickly as possible. A number of patients develop eye symptoms within four weeks of the onset of symptoms and it is essential to treat the condition at once if permanent disturbances of sight are to be avoided. Temporal arteritis is always associated with an increase in the red cell sedimentation rate in the blood. This is the rate at which red blood cells settle to the bottom of a narrow glass tube.

If you went to your doctor because you had symptoms which suggested that you might have temporal arteritis he might surprise you by taking your blood pressure in both of your arms and not only in one arm. This is because the disorder can affect arteries throughout the body, partially obstructing the blood flow in them. This could be detected by a difference in the readings of your blood pressure in your two arms. The doctor would also listen with his stethoscope along the course of major arteries for abnormal sounds which are called bruits. These are caused by changes in the vessel walls.

Temporal arteritis and polymyalgia rheumatica are usually self-limiting conditions and they tend to clear up over a period of 6 to 18 months. The vital thing is that the illness should be recognized as soon as possible and that treatment should be started immediately as this will prevent possible damage to eyesight. Patients with temporal arteritis usually respond to small doses of cortisone compounds, called steroids. For example 15 milligram a day of a drug called Prednisone might be enough in one patient while another patient might need 60 milligrams daily of the same drug. The treatment is tapered off gradually according to the improvement in headache symptoms and the way in which the blood sedimentation rate falls to, and remains at, normal levels. The pain of temporal arteritis often recedes rapidly when treatment is started.

If the diagnosis of temporal arteritis were in any doubt then a biopsy or small specimen could be taken from the wall of the temporal artery and examined under the microscope. This examination would reveal that part of the vessel wall had been destroyed and also show typical large cells, called giant cells. These changes in the blood vessel wall could extend to other arteries in the body, since the condition can affect any part of the arterial tree.

The course of temporal arteritis may extend over many months but it is usually a self-limiting disorder which clears up in time. Improvement is assessed by the lessening of symptoms and a fall in the raised red cell sedimentation rate to normal levels. The dosage of steroid therapy can be adjusted in accordance with the symptomatic improvement and the sedimentation rate.

CLUSTER HEADACHE

You will hardly be surprised by the fact that cluster headache is a headache that occurs in bouts or clusters. Opinions differ but it is generally considered to be a variety of migraine. It is one of those conditions where the diagnosis depends almost entirely on the story told by the sufferer. In 1822 Benjamin Hutchinson recorded a "hemicrania which after recurring for several hours daily for long periods — departs suddenly."

Unfortunately cluster headache has been given a number of names which tend to confuse the issue. Hence it is also recognised as Harris's periodic migrainous neuralgia, histamine headache, Horton's cephalgia. Horton provided the name cluster headache.

Eight times more men suffer from cluster headache than women. Some investigators have reported that cluster headache sufferers tend to drink and smoke more than average which will irritate those who do neither. Stomach ulcers are more common in cluster headache sufferers. The headaches can begin at any age but usually start between the ages of 30 and 40 years. Even a child of 5, however, has been reported as having cluster headache and it may start at the latter end of life. Reports also suggest that cluster headache is more common in the spring and autumn.

The story told by a sufferer from cluster headache is always typical. Sudden pain begins around one eye and rapidly becomes very severe. It may affect the same side of the head and neck and spread to the forehead and jaw. In desperate attempts to get rid of the pain the sufferer may throw himself around on the floor or bang his head against a wall. The eye on the painful side of the head often becomes pink and watery and the lid of the affected eye may droop. The nostril on the painful side may be blocked. The severe pain usually lasts a few minutes and then gradually wears off, but the poor victim is left dreading the next attack.

Six or more attacks may occur in a day and in some patients they arise with alarm clock regularity, waking the sufferer from sleep at precisely the same time each night, while the bouts persist. Sometimes the pain is relieved if the patient gets up and sits in a chair leaning forward with his head on his arms.

The headache spells may last for a few days or a few weeks and then disappear completely for days, months or even years. It seems very likely that the sensitivity of the blood vessels in the affected area is altered during the period of painful attacks. This is of great interest as provoking factors can induce an attack during the time when the vessels are sensitive whereas they will have no effect at all at another time. For example, patients who are suffering from a bout of cluster headaches will develop an attack within 30 to 50 minutes after taking a tablet containing one milligram of nitroglycerine under the tongue. (This is, of course, the same substance that is taken by patients suffering from angina and it relieves their pain because it causes blood vessels to dilate). Again, a substance called histamine, which is poured out in the tissues in response to shock or an allergic reaction, will in small doses produce an attack of cluster headache in a sufferer during a susceptible period. Alcohol is another substance to which sufferers from cluster headache are very sensitive during headache spells. We have only to think of the flushed face so readily produced by a glass or two of wine to realize that alcohol is a powerful dilator of superficial blood vessels. Alcohol should be strictly avoided during cluster headache episodes. Once the bout of headaches is over neither alcohol, nor histamine, nor nitroglycerine will have any headache-producing effect, and in any case one has to leave a latent period of a few hours from the last attack before a second one can be induced by any means.

Cluster headache is difficult to treat but fortunately the spell of attacks come to an end in the great majority of sufferers after a period of time. This obviously makes it hard to tell whether they have improved because of the treatment received or whether the bout of headaches has come to a natural conclusion.

During an attack of pain the blood vessels in the painful area enlarge and the pressure in the eye on the affected side of the head increases.

Ergotamine drugs are often successful because they cause the dilated blood vessels to constrict. Ergotamine can be taken in suppository form (1-2 mg) as effervescent tablets, or in an inhalant spray. Intramuscular ergotamine (0.25-0.5 mg) one hour before an expected attack may prove helpful.

Ergotamine has to be used with great caution as excess use of ergotamine can produce results worse than the original condition requiring treatment. When ergotamine compounds are being used in the treatment of cluster headache they should be discontinued completely every 7th day in order to find out whether or not the symptoms have abated.

Another drug which has been used in cluster headache is methysergide. This is given in 2 mg. doses four times a day. Treatment with ergotamine can be added at the end of a week if the methysergide alone is insufficient, but both ergotamine and methysergide can have unpleasant side effects which make it essential that they are used only under careful medical supervision.

Cortisone compounds have been tried in cluster headache and the results reported are promising. As soon as an attack begins the sufferer takes 30 mg. of Prednisone, often with almost immediate relief of pain. No more Prednisone may be needed as the single dose may be sufficient to abort the bout of attacks. If the suffer continues to get attacks then 20 mg. of Prednisone taken at breakfast time on every second day has been found to be helpful in diminishing their severity and frequency.

Lithium is another drug introduced more recently for the treatment of cluster headache. When this is used regular blood tests are essential as the level of lithium in the blood has to be maintained within certain levels (0.7 to 1.2 mmol/1).

During sleep all of us have rapid eye movements which are known by the abbreviation REM. They are symmetrical, jerky movements occurring several times during the average night's sleep, in spells of 5 to 60 minutes. They are associated with dreaming and in cluster headache sufferers are thought to be linked with the onset of a nocturnal bout of cluster headache. It is interesting to note that lithium which is used in cluster headache therapy reduces the incidence of rapid eye movements occurring during sleep.

Pizotifen is another drug that has been used with reported success in cluster headache in doses of 1.5 to 3.0 mg per day during bouts.

In 1978 a cluster headache sufferer wrote to an American medical journal that he had discovered a very successful method of dealing with his attacks. This was by inhaling oxygen. He stated that he used flowing oxygen at 10 liters a minute with a rebreathing bag mask and that this aborted his attacks in less than 10 minutes. Increased oxygen levels in the blood cause blood vessels to constrict which may be the main factor in its usefulness in this condition.

Occasionally, and certainly in not more than one in 10 cluster headache sufferers, the bouts of headaches persist throughout the year. Attempts to treat these patients surgically have failed to give encouraging results, but fortunately the advent of some of the newer drug therapies already mentioned are providing effective in allaying the symptoms.

TRIGEMINAL NEURALGIA

Before the days of antibiotics pneumonia was occasionally described as the friend of the very old. Gently and quietly it transported them from this world to the next. Equally graphically, trigeminal neuralgia was sometimes called the disorder which made an old person long for death. Trigeminal neuralgia is also known by the name of tic douloureux. This is because of the painful facial spasms or tics which sometimes accompany the excrutiatingly severe attacks of pain which characterize this complaint.

The nervous system consists of two parts. One part is called the autonomic nervous system which regulates those functions of which we are unaware and which are beyond our conscious control, such as the movement of the intestine. The other is the central nervous system which is made up of the brain and spinal cord and the nerves arising from them. The central nervous system controls voluntary movement and also receives sensory impulses. Thus the nerves arising from the brain and spinal cord are either motor nerves controlling voluntary movement or sensory nerves conveying sensations such as heat, pain and touch, or mixed nerves with both motor and sensory fibers.

Twelve pairs of nerves, called cranial nerves, arise from the brain and run chiefly to the head and neck. The fifth nerve is the largest of the cranial nerves and is called the trigeminal nerve. It is a mixed nerve containing motor and sensory fibers and has three main branches. The sensory fibers convey sensation from the face and forehead and the front of the chin. Roughly speaking the first part of the nerve conveys sensation from the forehead, eyelid and front of the nose, the second from the upper cheek, upper lip and nostril and the third from the side of the head and cheek around the front of the ear, chin and lower lip. It is this fifth cranial nerve which is involved in trigeminal neuralgia.

Trigeminal neuralgia rarely affects anyone under the age of 40 years. Women are affected twice as often as men and the pain is more frequently felt on the right side of the head than on the left. It usually starts in the second or third division of the nerve and therefore tends to affect the cheek and chin. The pain is very intense and occurs in brief bouts. It can be triggered off by such actions as chewing, talking or washing the face and has been described as feeling like red hot needles or an electric shock. The bouts of pain may occur over days, weeks or months with intervals of complete freedom. The patient with trigeminal neuralgia lives in dread of a recurrence of the symptoms although the outlook in this condition has improved greatly with advances in drug therapy. A drug called carbamazepine, for which the trade name is Tegretol, is effective in relieving the pain in the majority of sufferers from trigeminal neuralgia. This drug is usually given in doses of 200 mg three times a day, one hour before meals.

THE BLOOD SUPPLY OF THE HEAD

Volume for volume the head is the heaviest part of the body. The weight of the head is reduced a little by virtue of the fact that it contains a number of air pockets or sinuses. The bones of the head can be separated into the skull which contains the brain and the bones of the face. The skull forms a solid case protecting the brain which is a relatively soft organ. The brain is wrapped in three tissue paper like sheaths called meninges, and cushioned by a thin layer of fluid, the cerebro-spinal fluid, which circulates between them. This fluid acts as a buffer between the brain and spinal cord on the one hand and the bones of the skull and backbone which provide a solid frame for them. The cerebrospinal fluid acts as a shock absorber and its composition and pressure are regulated by a very delicate mechanism.

Because the skull is rigid, the space within it is strictly limited and pain results from any sudden change in intracranial pressure. Such a change could result from an increase or decrease in the volume of cerebrospinal fluid. For example, in meningitis, which is an inflammation of the sheaths wrapped around the brain, the volume of fluid increases and headaches occur.

In a lumbar puncture a small hollow needle is inserted between the third and fourth lumbar vertebrae of the spine and a few drops of cerebrospinal fluid are removed. This investigation reveals whether or not the fluid is under increased pressure, whether its composition is normal and whether or not any infection is present.

The average brain weighs 1400 grams. Curiously enough the brains of women weigh a few grams less than those of men. In an adult at rest the heart pumps out approximately 5.6 litres of blood per minute. The brain is supplied with nearly a litre of blood every minute which means that in an individual at rest the brain receives roughly 15 to 20% of the total output of blood from the heart. The blood supply to the brain remains remarkably constant even in fairly extreme circumstances.

In 1783 a scientist called Munro stated that because the brain was enclosed inside the rigid casing of the skull and could not be compressed, the quantity of blood in the head could not alter. Munro therefore concluded that the blood vessels supplying the brain, unlike other blood vessels in the body, were passive and incapable of changing in size. This, however, is not true. The blood vessels of the brain are richly supplied with nerves which carefully and intricately regulate their size and maintain a constant blood flow. Consciousness is not lost until the blood flow falls below 32 c.c. per 100 grams of brain per minute which is less than half the normal flow. Irreversible brain damage occurs if the flow is less than 10 c.c. per 100 grams of brain tissue per minute.

The brain is unique, because it is supplied by no less than three main arteries. These are the two carotid arteries and the basilar artery.

The carotid arteries can be felt, and sometimes seen beating on either side of the neck. Each of the carotid arteries divides into an internal carotid branch which runs into the inside of the skull and an external carotid artery which supplies blood chiefly on the outside of the skull. Running up the backbone, on either side of the spinal cord are the vertebral arteries. The vertebral arteries join together at the base of the skull to form the single basilar artery. The basilar artery joins with branches from the two internal carotid arteries to form a highly efficient arterial circuit at the base of the brain. This arterial circuit, first described by Thomas Willis is known as the circle of Willis. It ensures that even if one part of the blood supply to the brain is blocked for any reason the brain will still receive an adequate blood supply through the rest of the circuit.

Outside the skull or cranium, that is on the outside of the head, the blood supply is provided by the external carotid artery on each side of the head.

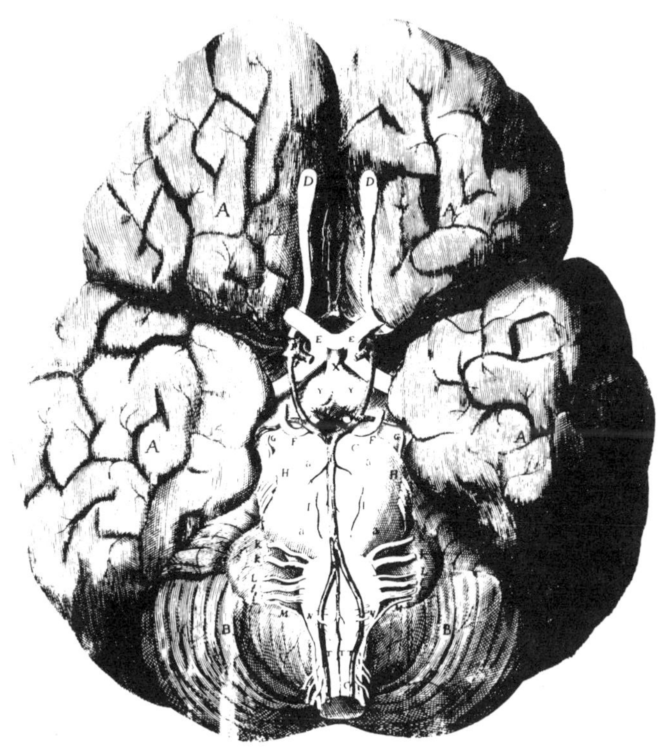

The Circle of Willis

It is obviously essential that the centres in the brain which control vital functions in the body such as the heart beat and breathing should receive an adequate blood supply. Unlike the cells in muscle, nerve cells have no stores of glucose to call upon in an emergency. They are dependent on the nutrients carried to them by the blood. Oxygen is essential to the life of cells in the human body and this too is carried in the red cells of the blood.

The main factor regulating the blood flow to the brain appears to be the carbon dioxide content of the air that we breathe. Normally this is around 0.04% but if it is raised to 7% then the blood flow to the brain is doubled. Conversely, a reduction in the carbon dioxide level in the blood supplying the brain results in a decrease in flow.

The response to the effect of carbon dioxide lessens with increasing age. This is hardly surprising as one might expect blood vessels to become increasingly rigid and less responsive with age. Neither sleep nor concentrated mental effort have any effect on brain blood flow. A severe drop in body temperature reduces the flow but this may be because the cooler body uses less oxygen and thus produces less carbon dioxide.

There are obvious difficulties in trying to discover what is happening to the blood flow in the brain of man. During the last 30 years, however, techniques have been developed which enable this to be done. Originally these techniques were based on the Fick principle. The Fick principle states that the blood flow to any organ can be measured by determining the amount of a given substance (Qx) removed from the blood stream by the organ per unit of time, and dividing that value by the difference between the concentration of the substance in arterial blood (Ax) and venous blood (Vx) going to and returning from the organ.

Thus to determine the cerebral blood flow (CBF) one would use the formula

$$CBF = \frac{Qx}{Ax - Vx}$$

Nitrous oxide was one of the earliest substances used in attempts to determine the blood flow to the brain by this method.

Subsequently radioactive gas clearance techniques were developed and the gamma emissions of radioactive substances such as $Xenon_{133}$ were counted. The snag is that any inhalation method of determining blood flow in the head means that the substance being measured leaves the lungs and is distributed in the areas supplied by both the internal and external carotid arteries. The figures thus obtained reflect the blood flow in the vessels both inside and outside the skull. Since we are particularly interested in what is going on inside the skull a search has been made for new methods that will provide this information. Radioactive materials have been injected directly into the internal carotid artery and the gamma emissions counted as in the earlier method of inhalation. This time, however, they reflect the flow of blood in the area supplied by the internal carotid artery only and thus tells us more about what is going on inside the skull.

Thermography

When the blood flow to an area is increased then the temperature of the skin over the area rises. Thermography is a technique by which changes in skin temperature can be recorded. It is possible to obtain a visual record of this heat production and this is called a thermogram. Tumor tissue, for example, emits more heat than normal tissue and thermography has been used in screening programs to detect very early cases of breast cancer. Thermography has been used to show changes in blood flow in the painful area of the head during migraine attacks and has also revealed "cold" spots, usually around the eyes, in patients suffering from cluster headache.

THE BLOOD BRAIN BARRIER

Paul Ehrlich was not a brilliant boy at school and he hated examinations but he became one of the greatest pioneers in medicine and science. He was born in Poland in 1854 and 54 years later was awarded the Nobel Prize in Medicine, jointly with Ilya Mechnikov for work on immunity. Paul Ehrlich was particularly interested in the way in which synthetic dyes affected living tissues and concentrated on methods of staining cells in the blood. His original work in this area led to him being regarded as the founder of modern haematology which is the study of the blood, and he introduced new techniques in many other areas of medicine. For example, he stained the tubercle bacillus so that it could be clearly identified under a microscope and he developed methods for standardizing antisera like diptheria antitoxin which are still in use today. Ehrlich also made great advances in drug therapy. However, there is a particular reason for thinking about him in connection with headaches.

Ehrlich was the first person to demonstrate that when basic dyes are injected into the blood stream they reach the tissue of the brain, whereas acidic dyes, like trypan blue, fail to stain the grey matter The fact that only certain dyes stain brain tissue suggests that there is a barrier which prevents some substances from reaching the brain. This barrier is called the blood brain barrier. It cannot be seen or identified but the hypothetical idea of a barrier between the blood and the brain is helpful when we try to understand the actions of various drugs. We know, for example, that substances which dissolve in fat can cross the blood brain barrier, while those which are water soluble fail to do so. Not surprisingly, potent pain relieving drugs and volatile anaesthetics are fat soluble.

There is one small area of the brain where the barrier appears to be defective. This is in a part of the brain called the hypothalamus, and it is possible that some substances, which would be prevented from gaining access to the brain by the blood brain barrier, manage to get through this unprotected gap.

The concept of a blood brain barrier is important when we think about the various types of headaches and the way in which these arise. It will be mentioned again in the relevant sections in this book.

WHAT IS MIGRAINE?

How can you tell that you are suffering from migraine and not just from ordinary headaches? The term migraine is often loosely used, possibly because it used to be thought that migraine affected only the more intelligent members of the population! It is certainly true that some of the best accounts of migraine attacks have been given by philosophers and astronomers but this is because they form an articulate section of the population and not because migraine selects its victims according to their mental abilities. So how could you arrive at a diagnosis of migraine? Well, to start with, migraine is a headache which recurs at intervals. So, of course, do other types of headache. Migraine sufferers, however, often get a warning that a headache is about to begin. These warning symptoms take many forms and are collectively termed prodromal symptoms or an "aura". Thus one migraine sufferer may become aware of an impending attack when part of the page of the book he is reading becomes blotted out. Another may notice bright spots coming and going before his eyes or flashing lights. Less commonly tingling is felt in an arm or a leg, and limpness or loss of power may occur in a small proportion of patients. These symptoms usually last about 20 minutes and then the headache begins. In a very small number of migraine sufferers the prodromal symptoms do not lead to headache symptoms on all, or even in rare instances on any, occasions. These people learn to accept their occasional symptoms as warnings of a possible attack which will not necessarily follow.

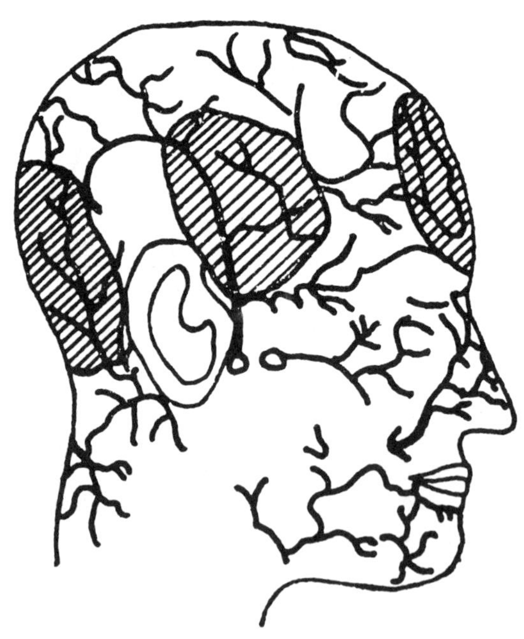

Common Sites of Pain in Migraine.

Lewis Carroll suffered severely from migraine. Possibly he was describing his own prodromal symptoms or aura when telling us how Alice in Wonderland felt as her body grew larger and larger and her head distorted in size after she had followed the White Rabbit down the rabbit hole and eaten the small cake marked "Eat me". Some migraine sufferers feel extra cheerful or energetic in the few hours preceding an attack. The commonest prodromal symptoms, however, affect eyesight and some of the best descriptions of these visual symptoms have been recorded by astronomers. One of these accounts was given by George Biddell Airy. Airy was born in 1801 and by the time that he was 17 his tutor in mathematics had to give him notice as the pupil had outshone his teacher! Airy subsequently excelled at Cambridge where he was able to achieve a degree of financial independence by coaching students in his own class. After such an auspicious beginning to his career we can hardly be surprised to learn that he became a Professor at the age of 26.

In 1834 Airy was elected Astronomer Royal, an appointment which he held for 46 years. He is particularly remembered for discovering the way in which lenses can be used to correct astigmatism. Airy has left us an account of the visual symptoms which he experienced with his attacks of migraine, and after describing the zig zag shapes which formed arches in front of his eyes, he pondered "I have never been able to decide with certainty whether the disease really affects both eyes. The impression on the mind is that only one eye is affected. There is general obscurity on one side, but the tremor and boiling are so oppressive, that, if produced only in one eye, they may nearly extinguish the corresponding vision in the other.

The duration of the ocular derangement with me is usually from twenty to thirty minutes, but with one of my friends it sometimes last much longer. In general I feel no further inconvenience from it; but with my friends it is followed by an oppressive headache. In one instance it was remarked that the mouth of a person afflicted was sensibly distorted on one side. And in one attack on myself, which occurred while I was conversing with an acquaintance in a railway carriage, I soon became painfully sensible that I had not the usual command of speech, that my memory failed so much that I did not know what I had said or had attempted to say, and I might be talking incoherently."

Airy concludes this account by expressing his views.

"I entertain no doubt that the seat of the disease is the brain, that the disease is a species of paralysis, and that the occular affection is only a secondary symptom."

Volumes have been written about the visual prodromata of migraine. They usually last about 15 to 20 minutes and then the pain begins. This often affects one side of the head more than the other and can become extremely severe, so severe in fact that the sufferer has to retreat to bed and the least effort, such as coughing, or even raising the head from the pillow, intensifies the pain. Nausea and vomiting frequently accompany the headache. The whole attack may be over in a few hours or last a whole day. In between attacks the migraine sufferer is headache free. The pain persists in roughly one in ten migraine sufferers who also suffer from tension headache. Migraine tends to run in families. Very careful studies by Danish investigators have revealed that when patients with migraine from different families are questioned over 90% of them give a history of migraine in other members of their family. Similar studies were undertaken in London.

When 500 migraine sufferers were asked whether other members of their families suffered from headaches, over 60% of them gave a family history of migraine in one or other parent. It was twice as common in the mothers of these patients as in the fathers.

So we can draw up a list of features which distinguish migraine from other types of headache.

1. Migraine tends to run in families.

2. Attacks recur at intervals between which the sufferer is usually free of headache.

3. Warning symptoms occur in a proportion of patients. These are usually visual.

4. The headache is often accompanied by a feeling of nausea, and sometimes vomiting.

5. The pain of a migraine attack often affects one side of the head more than the other.

ABDOMINAL MIGRAINE

This is a rare variant of migraine in which the attacks of pain in the head are replaced by recurrent attacks of abdominal pain. This pain may be associated with nausea and vomiting and it is only its recurrence in the absence of

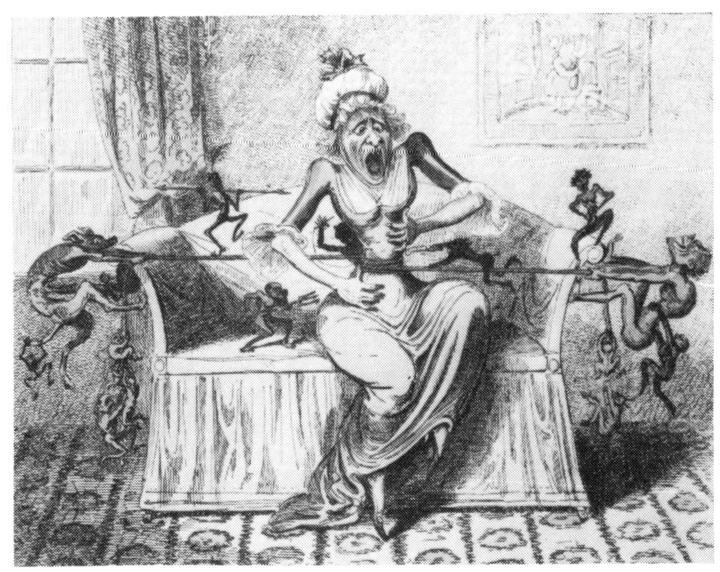

The Cholic

any abnormal physical findings, in a patient with a family history of migraine, that eventually leads the physician to the correct diagnosis. Like migraine in childhood it is a diagnosis which can only be arrived at by a process of exclusion. Abdominal migraine is interesting in so far as the symptoms appear to respond more readily to anticonvulsant therapy, than to other drugs usually used in the treatment of migraine.

WHAT HAPPENS IN A MIGRAINE ATTACK?

During an attack of migraine a number of changes occur in the size of blood vessels in the head. Two stages are recognised. During the prodromal or first phase of an attack there is a narrowing in some of the branches of the internal carotid artery.

The only way in which blood vessels can be viewed directly in the intact body is by means of an instrument called an ophthalmoscope. With this instrument a light is shone through the pupil on to the back of the eye which can then be inspected through a magnifying lens. At the back of the eye is the retina which is the part of the eye sensitive to light. Across the retina are the fine terminal branches of the optic nerve which transmit the impulses from the retina to the centres in the brain which are responsible for interpreting vision. The head of the optic nerve is seen as a flat white disc, the optic disc, on the retina. Across the retina runs a network of arteries and veins, and by examining these one can obtain a good idea of the general state of the blood vessels in the body. For example in a patient with a high blood pressure changes occur at an early stage in the blood vessels of the retina. Changes are found in some patients with diabetes and in a large number of other disorders. Thus an examination of the retina with an ophthalmoscope is a helpful routine part of a medical examination.

The blood vessels on the retina have been observed during the prodromal stage of a migraine attack. This is the time during which the sufferer from classical migraine complains of warning symptoms such as visual disturbances. Examination of the eyes with an ophthalmoscope has confirmed that during this phase the retinal vessels on both sides of the head become narrowed. In fact the blood flow in the internal carotid artery may be reduced to half its previous level.

The blood vessels in the cerebral circulation are extremely sensitive to changes in the oxygen and carbon dioxide content of the blood. A rise in carbon dioxide levels causes a dilation of the cerebral blood vessels. It is interesting to note that the prodromal symptoms of migraine are sometimes relieved when the sufferer breathes in and out of a paper bag. This simple measure increases the carbon dioxide content of the blood and causes the cerebral vessels to dilate.

The prodromal phase of migraine during which constriction of the vessels takes place is followed by a stage in which the vessels on the side of the head on which pain develops become enlarged and throbbing. The vessels affected at this stage are the branches of the external carotid artery and these dilated, throbbing branches can often be seen standing out on the side of the head in the painful area. Some of the branches of the external carotid artery pass through the skull bone to the inside of the head and the pain of migraine is probably due chiefly to the distension of these vessels.

The changes in the size of blood vessels which accompany an attack of migraine are associated with a number of biochemical changes. These have been mentioned in the section of this book dealing with the chemistry of migraine. One of the vasoactive amines concerned in these changes is 5-hydroxytryptamine. This amine is also concerned with pain production, and is mentioned in more detail in the section of this book dealing with pain.

MEDICAL TREATMENT AND MIGRAINE

*"... when Moses made a brazen serpent and set it up
on a staff, the wounded men had but to look towards it
and they were healed."*

Numbers, Ch. 21, v.9.

Until the time of Hippocrates the art of healing was a branch of magic or religion. Prior to Hippocrates, the Greek Aesculapius dominated the scene. Later worshipped as the god of healing, he is a shadowy semi-mythical figure who may have existed in approximately 1250 B.C. Legend tells us that he had great healing powers and even restored the dead to life. Because of this Pluto, the king of the underworld, became resentful as he felt that he was losing too many new recruits to his kingdom and he appealed to Zeus to intervene. Zeus responded by slaying Aesculapius with a thunderbolt. From the time of his death Aesculapius was worshipped as a god and temples to him were erected all over Greece, notably in Athens, Pergamos and Epidaurus. There was also a temple to Aesculapius at Cos.

Sick people came to these temples to be healed by the ritual of incubation. When the sick person arrived at the temple he first offered a sacrifice to the god. He purified

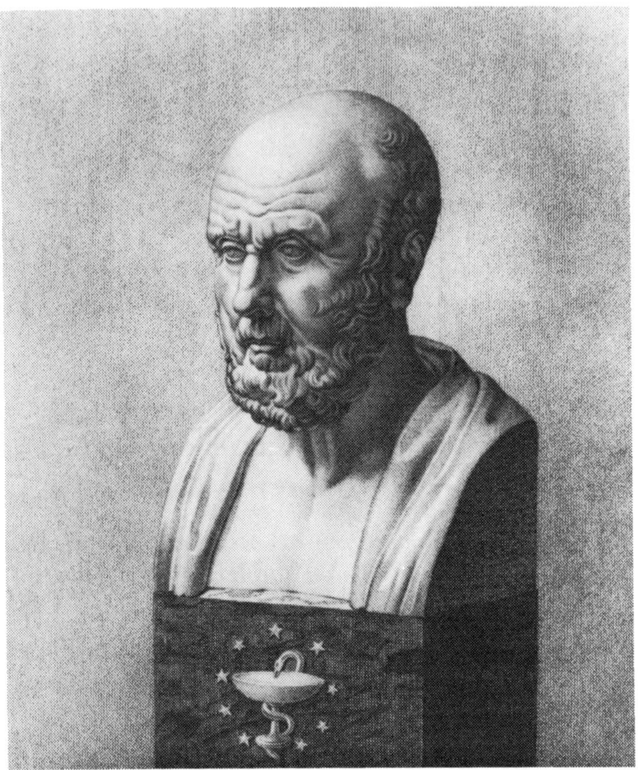

Hippocrates.

himself by bathing, and then lay down to sleep in the abaton or long colonnade. This stretched along the side of the temple and was open to the air. During the night the god Aesculapius was supposed to appear to the supplicant in a dream and to give advice and treatment. In the morning those patients who had benefitted from their visit left the temple. Others remained sometimes for long periods of time. We are told that while the sick were sleeping in the temples of Aesculapius their eyes or sores were licked by the harmless snakes that were common in Greece. The snakes were believed to assist in the process of healing, and the serpent is still a symbol of healing today. It is incorporated in the insignia of many military and non-military medical organizations in the world.

We know about the ritual of healing or incubation in the temples of Aesculapius because of the inscriptions on stone tablets found at Epidaurus. This was the site of the god's most famous shrine. Aesculapius himself was said to be the son of Apollo, the sun god. Legend has it that Aesculapius had two daughters with the rather mundane names of Hygieia (the Greek word for health) and Panacea (meaning cure). Hippocrates, the father of medicine is reputed to be a descendant of one of these daughters. Hippocrates was born in 460 B.C. on the island of Cos, close to the coast of Asia Minor. A living relic supposedly of his time is the huge oriental plane tree which stands in the centre of Cos. It was under these branches, now supported from every angle, that Hippocrates is thought to have lectured to his students in the open air. He was the first to insist on careful observation and the interpretation of symptoms and was convinced that disease resulted from natural and not supernatural causes.

Hippocrates introduced method into medicine and it is the oath of Hippocrates which has been sworn by generations of medical students when they obtain their final qualification. This oath laid down clear guide lines for the highest standards of medical practice and one might reflect with sorrow on the way in which part of it is being abused today in relation to the sanctity of human life.

The Hippocratic Oath states in full,

> I swear by Apollo the physician and Aesculapius and health and all heal, (that is by Hygieia and Panacea) and all the Gods and Goddesses, that according to my ability and judgement I will keep this oath and this stipulation to reckon him who taught me this Art equally dear to me as my Parents, to share my substance with him and relieve his necessities if required, to look upon his offspring in the same footing as my own brothers, and to teach them this Art if they shall wish to learn it, without fee or stipulation. And that by precept, lecture and every other mode of Instruction, I will impart a knowledge of the Art

to my own Sons, and those of my Teachers, and to Disciples bound by a stipulation and Oath according to the Law of Medicine. But to none others. I will follow that system of regimen, which according to my Ability and Judgement, I consider for the benefit of my patients, and abstain from whatever is deleterious and mischievous. I will give no deadly Medicine to anyone if asked, nor suggest any such Counsel. And in like manner I will not give to a Woman a Pessary to procure Abortion. With Purity and with Holiness I will pass my life and practise my Art. I will not cut persons labouring under the stone but will leave this to be done by men who are Practitioners of this work. Into whatever houses I enter I will go into them for the benefit of the sick, and will abstain from every voluntary act of mischief and corruption, and further from the Seduction of Females or Males or Freemen and Slaves. Whatever, in connection with my professional practice or not in connection with it, I see or hear in the life of men which ought not to be spoken of abroad, I will not divulge, as reckoning that all such should be kept secret. While I continue to keep this Oath unviolated, may it be granted to me to enjoy life and the practice of the Art, respected by all men in all times. But should I trespass and violate this Oath, may the reverse be my lot.

The oath begins "I swear by Apollo". Apollo was god of the sun and god of the intellect and is associated with two basic Greek precepts which every migraine sufferer would do well to reflect upon. These are "Know thyself" and "Nothing in excess". Greek culture respected the value of the individual in society and it is this basic understanding of human nature that makes so many of the writings of the philosophers of ancient Greece as applicable now as they were in their own day.

The hellenistic Greeks extended the advances in knowledge made by Hippocrates, particularly in the sphere of anatomy as they dissected the bodies of dead criminals. The Romans were more practical. They accepted Greek philosophies and in particular the arguments of Zeno of Cyprus (336—264 B.C.), who considered that the greatest good in life was to become indifferent to sorrow, pleasure, and pain. In opposition to this stoic philosophy the skeptics argued that no two people could agree on absolute values of sorrow, pleasure and pain and that the wise man steers his course along a middle way while accepting the customs of his day and time. The more practical nature of the Romans led them to institute the first hospitals. They also introduced hydrotherapy which is the use of mineral water baths for healing purposes. This emphasis by the Romans on the use of water can be regarded as one of the earliest steps in the promotion of public health measures.

Migraine was described by the Greek physician Galen who lived from A.D. 130 to 200. Galen was the greatest anatomist and physiologist of classical times and ranked highest as a brain and nerve anatomist. He was born at Pergamum and was surgeon to the gladiators there which no doubt gave him ample opportunity to link clinical observations with anatomical structure. He later became physician to the Emperor Marcus Aurelius and was the first to feel the pulse as an aid to diagnosis. He was a careful observer and a prolific writer. Of migraine he said:

> "Hemicrania is a painful disorder affecting approximately one half of the head, either the right or the left side, and which extends along the length of the longitudinal suture . . . It is caused by the ascent of vapours, either excessive in amount, or too hot, or too cold."

Galen was the founder of experimental physiology. After he introduced the term hemicrania it was gradually modified through hemigrania, emigranea, migranea, megrim to its present form migraine. Galen wrote a medical encyclopedia which remained the standard reference book for medical men until the Renaissance.

Between the years 900 to 1100 A.D. muslim learning

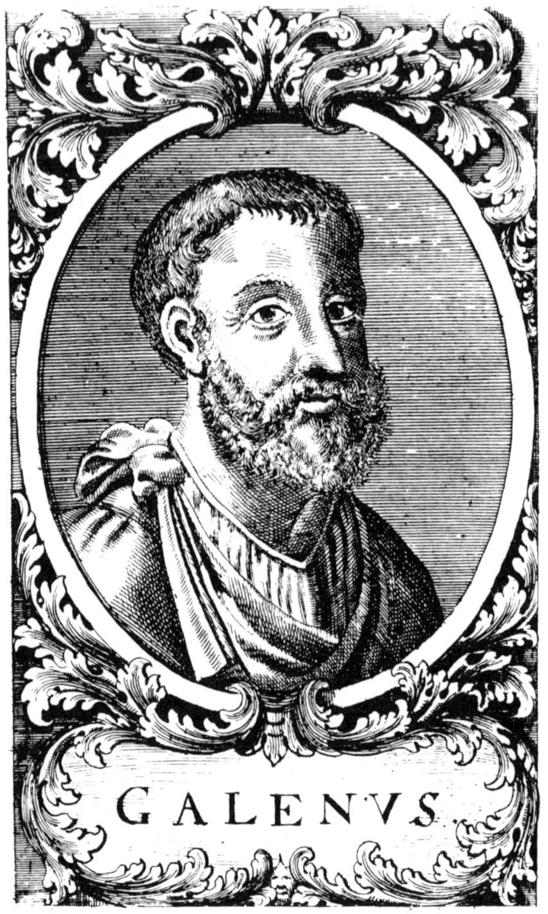

Galen 130-200 A.D.

made great contributions to medicine and a comprehensive encyclopedia incorporating all aspects of medical knowledge to that date was compiled by a Persian physician and alchemist of Baghdad called Rhazes.

The first complete and illustrated book on Surgery and Instruments was written by Albucasis, an Arabian surgeon, who died in A.D. 1013. A beautifully produced definitive edition of the Arabic text with an English translation by Dr. M.S. Spink and Dr. G.L. Lewis has been published by the Wellcome Institute of the History of Medicine. The method described by Albucasis for the relief of migraine evokes thoughts of torture rather than treatment. But let me quote from this monumental translation of Albucasis and you can judge for yourselves.

When there occurs pain with headache in one side of the head and the pain extends to the eye; and the patient has cleared his head with purging drugs and there has been applied the other treatment that I have mentioned in the sections on diseases, but to no avail; in this disorder cauterisation is of two sorts, either with caustic or with the actual cautery. This is the manner of cauterisation with caustic; take one clove of garlic; peel it and cut both ends off; then cut open the site of the pain in the temple with a broad scalpel till there is room to contain the clove under the skin; then introduce it under the skin till it lies completely hidden. Then bind up the wound tightly over it with pads and leave for fifteen hours; then unbind it, remove the garlic and leave the wound open for two or three days; then apply cotton wool soaked in butter till it suppurates. Then dress with ointment till it heals . . .

The actual cauterisation with iron should be done in this way: heat a cautery of this shape. It is called the claviform; the head is nail-shaped in that there is a slight curvature with a small protuberance in the middle. Apply it then to the site of the pain, hold your hand steady and revolve it little by little. Let the thickness of skin burnt be about half; then remove your hand so as not to burn a subjacent artery, for thus a haemorrhage arises. Then soak some cotton wool in saline, apply to the place, and leave three days; then apply cotton wool with butter; then treat with ointment till it heals. Or if you prefer you can cauterize this migraine with the knife-edge that juts out from the cautery, but be careful not to cut an artery, specially in this kind of migraine that is non-chronic.

When you have treated a migraine in the way we have described and with what we have mentioned in the sections on diseases, and the treatment is ineffective, and you perceive that the malady is such that the cauterization we have mentioned before does not suffice for it, either with caustic or with the actual artery, you should heat an edged cautery to white heat after you have marked the place with a line half a finger's breadth long or thereabouts; and impress your hand once and maintain the pressure till you cut down upon the artery and reach the bone. You must be careful of the mandibular joint which moves in chewing, that you do not cut the muscle or tendon that moves it, causing spasm. Have the utmost care of haemorrhage from the artery you have cut, for the occurrence of that is dangerous, specially with one who does not know what to do, having no experience or practice; it is better to refrain from operating. We shall later on mention a treatment for accidental haemorrhage of the artery, in due detail, in its proper place in this book. But if you see that this cautery is not enough for this disorder and you see that the patient is of bodily fitness for it, cauterize him in the middle of the head as we have described, and treat the wound till healed."

The author mentions that Hippocrates advocated bleeding for chronic headache and that Celsus who gave us the classic description of inflammation also described cauterization of the temporal veins.

When the measures already described by Albucasis failed extraction of the temporal arteries was recommended. This was undertaken as follows:

"The manner of extraction is for the patient to shave the temporal hair; then you press upon the artery appearing on the temple; for it will be manifest to you by its pulsation, and is rarely invisible save in a few people or on account of severe cold. But if it is not plain to you then let the patient bind his neck with the end of his garment; then do you rub the place with a piece of cloth or forment with hot water, till the artery is obvious to you; then take a scalpel shaped thus then with it gently scrape away the skin till you come to the artery, then stick a hook in it and draw it upwards till you extract it from the skin and free it all round from the membranes that are beneath it. But if the artery be thin, twist it with the tip of the hook and cut out enough of it for the two ends to be well separated from one another and contrast so that no haemorrhage occurs; for if it is not divided and cut it will not let blood flow at all. Then let blood, from six to three counces."

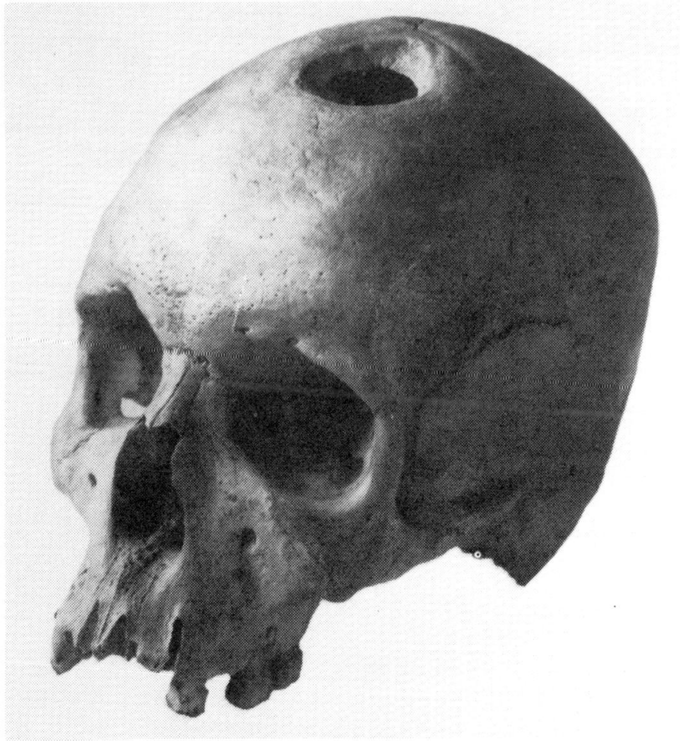

A Trephined Skull.

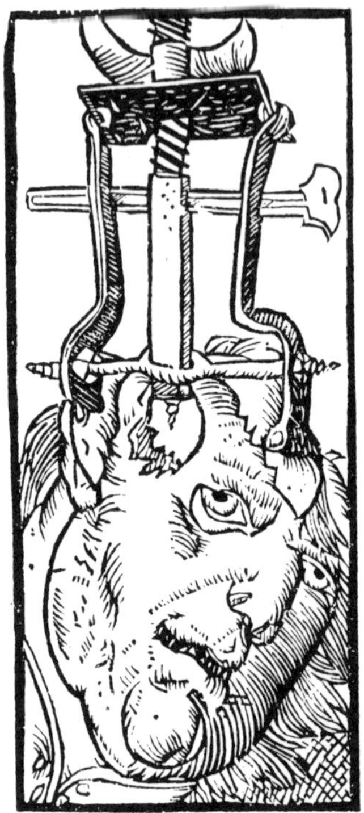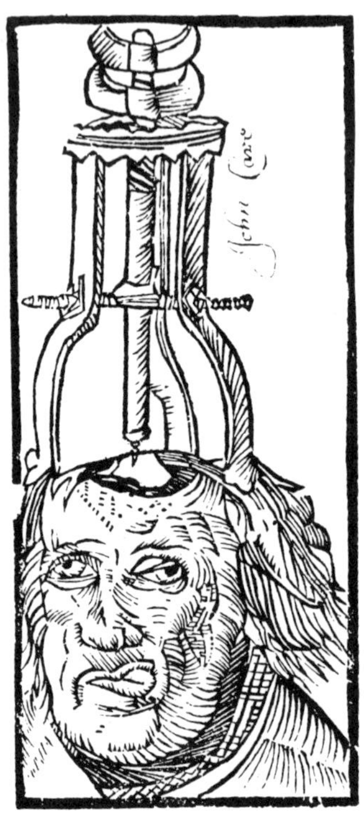

Trephining of the skull, early 16th century.

Bleeding from veins was also undertaken and provides us with our last graphic description taken from the translation of Albucasis.

"Venesection of the two veins behind the ears. Bleeding from both of these will give relief in cases of chronic catarrh, migraine and chronic foul pustules, and scabs of the head. The method of venesecting these two is as I shall now describe; the patient's head should be shaved and the hinder part, in the region of the two veins, should be strongly chafed with a rough cloth; then the patient should bind his neck with his turban until the two veins are visible; their position is behind the ears in the two flattened places of the head; feel for them with your fingers and when you feel their pulsation beneath your finger then mark the place with ink. Then take a knife scalpel, known as a lancet, and insert it beneath the vessel into the skin until the scalpel reaches the bone; then lifting with your hand both vessel and skin make an incision dividing both skin and vein; the length of the incision should be about two fingers side by side; then draw off the quantity of blood you wish. Then bind them up with dressings and leave it until healed."

The fact that patients were prepared to undergo such drastic treatment is some indication of the suffering from which they were seeking relief. Fortunately the passing of a thousand years has provided us with less violent remedies.

It was during the last fifteenth and sixteenth centuries that medicine was put on a truly scientific basis.

In 1493 Aureolus Philippus Theophrastus Bombastus von Hohenheim was born at Einsiedeln in Switzerland. His fourth name appears to have described his character fairly well but he gave himself the name of Paracelsus. He was the son of a physician who taught him physics and surgery and at the age of 16 he went to the University of Basle, where he subsequently became town physician. Captivated by the study of chemistry and alchemy he thought that he had discovered the secret of the philosophers stone. He also thought that by using an elixir that he had made he would reach the age of Methuselah. Paracelsus advocated experimental science and taught that since the human body is composed largely of chemical material then chemicals should be used to treat human disease. He was a great believer in the influence of the stars and his views subsequently had a considerable impact on the thinking of Franz Mesmer. Paracelsus disputed the teachings of Hippocrates and Galen and his aggressive, arrogant manner made him many enemies. He is said to have drunk too much and seldom changed his clothes and despite his faith in his Elixir he died at the early age of 48 years. His influence on medical thought was profound.

While Paracelsus was preaching the importance of chemistry in medical treatment, Andreas Vesalius, a native of Brussels was preparing his great work on Anatomy "The Fabric of the Human Body". This was published in 1543, and greatly advanced the understanding of anatomy and in particular the understanding of the nervous system. At about the same time William Harvey (1578-1657) was achieving for physiological science what Vesalius had done for anatomy. In 1628 he published his celebrated treatise "Exercitatio Anatomica de Motu Cordis et Sanguinis", in which he expounded his views on the circulation of the blood. About 80 years later Stephen Hales, who studied at Corpus Christi College Cambridge and became a perpetual curate at Teddington near London, was the first to make direct blood pressure recordings. He did this in a horse by inserting a hollow tube into the carotid artery in the neck and observing the level to which the column of blood rose. The importance of his findings remained unrecognized until the end of the nineteenth century.

Further major advances in medicine were the introduction of human vaccination for smallpox around 1787 by Edward Jenner, the introduction of aseptic techniques by Joseph Lister in 1860 and the demonstration in the second half of the nineteenth century by Louis Pasteur and Robert Koch, that germs were responsible for diseases.

At about the same time, in fact just over 100 years ago, a surgeon, Mr. J.H. Walsh, published a book on Domestic medicine and Surgery [1] in which he divided headache into four categories, rheumatic, congestive, dyspeptic and periodic. Migraine was included with the dyspeptic type of headache. Measures such as the wearing of a flannel cap sprinkled with camphorated spirit of wine were advocated for "rheumatic" headache, while cupping and the application of leeches were recommended for "congestive" headache. The author was less hopeful about the treatment of sick headache or migraine. He wrote "In sickheadache however, which is generally confined to the first half of life very little can be done by any means, and the only consolation which can be afforded is, that in course of time the attacks gradually disappear. Large doses of quinine have been found to keep them off for a time, but at-last they have failed in every case where I have known them tried. Aperients seem to be wholly useless, and, indeed, it may be said that the resources of medicine have been tried in vain."

Fortunately the resources of the twentieth century have brought enormous therapeutic advances in medicine. Today we have a large number of drugs available for the treatment of migraine; but before seeking any treatment at all every migraine sufferer should take to heart the two words of wisdom inscribed on the walls of the most famous temple of Apollo at Delphi in ancient Greece. There is written "Know thyself".

The common causes of migraine are stress, hormonal factors, dietary factors and fasting.

Stress covers a wide field of precipitating causes ranging from the excitement of a visit to the theatre to the anxiety of wondering whether or not the gas tap was turned off at the oven. If you are a migraine sufferer then probably the easiest way to discover why your migraine attacks occur when they do is by keeping a record of them over a period of time. A minimum period of at least three months is advisable. If you have a pocket diary it is easy to jot down when you get a headache and to note any associated factors that could have played a part in causing it. Women should record the dates of menstrual periods as the hormonal cycle sometimes bears a relation to the incidence of headache. This fact may not be immediately apparent. Headaches often occur midway between two monthly periods, and it is only when a careful record is kept that the link gradually becomes evident. A note should also be made of any possible dietary factors that could be relevant, such as the eating of chocolate or taking of alcoholic drinks. Similarly you should note if you missed a meal or if any other circumstances arose that might have contributed to your headache. Only you can know what these factors might be as they vary so much from one person to another.

We are all individuals and migraine sufferers must remember that it is only as individuals that they can hope to work out what the contributing causes to their headaches may be. For example, constipation or the taking of excessive laxatives can both be aggravating factors during a spell of recurring headaches.

Having tried to ascertain as far as possible whether or not any particular factors are associated with attacks, the migraine sufferer, with the help of his or her doctor, can then try to counteract them as far as possible. The treatment of migraine can be considered in two parts, firstly preventive or prophylactic treatment and then therapy for the acute attack.

Prophylactic therapy

Emphasis has already been placed on the most important prophylactic therapy which lies in understanding the common causes of migraine. This alone can lead to a considerable reduction in the number and severity of attacks. As already stated the most commonly cited precipitant of migraine attacks is stress.

It is not always possible to avoid occasions which cause stress and for this reason the use of a mild sedative is occasionally helpful to the migraine sufferer. If you know that you are going to get very anxious about an interview, or that you will find a particular journey worrying it will probably make all the difference if you take the edge off it with the help of a tablet from your doctor. Of course it would be quite wrong to rely on sedatives as a routine aid to daily living but to illustrate the point, the old proverb of a stitch in time saves nine, might well be translated into a medical context. Some of the drugs used specifically for the prophylaxis of migraine contain a mild sedative for this reason. Valium, in doses of 2 mg three times a day may be helpful for a period of a few weeks in a migraine sufferer whose attacks have been severe and frequent and clearly related to stress. A mild sedative at night, ensuring sound sleep and relaxation may also be beneficial.

There are a number of drugs on the market which have been used specifically in migraine prophylaxis.

Methysergide Therapy

Normal blood contains a substance called 5-hydroxytryptamine. This is also called serotonin and can be abbreviated to 5HT. At the onset of a migraine attack the level of this substance falls to about forty per cent of its usual level. The role of 5HT in migraine has been extensively investigated and about eighty per cent of migraine sufferers investigated have shown this drop in 5HT levels at the onset of an attack. It seems reasonable, therefore, to assume that a change in 5HT levels is a feature of migraine attacks.

Soon after it was established that the levels of 5HT in the blood played a role in the migraine attack, the drug methysergide was introduced into migraine therapy. Methysergide acts as a powerful antagonist of 5HT and has proved to be an effective preventive treatment in migraine. It lessens the frequency and the severity of attacks in well over half the sufferers in whom it has been used.

Unfortunately, however, there are snags. Methysergide is not without possible harmful effects. These usually begin to occur after treatment with the drug has been given for several weeks and the incidence is thought to be about forty per cent. All drugs have certain toxic effects in common and these, as one might expect, are nausea, vomiting and diarrhea. Skin rashes are also a common toxic effect of most drugs. These relatively mild toxic side effects may be accompanied by nervousness and insomnia in patients on methysergide treatment. The mild mental effects produced occasionally may have some bearing on the fact that methysergide is chemically related to the psychotropic drug LSD. About fifteen per cent of the patients on methysergide therapy have to discontinue treatment with the drug because of these side effects.

Methysergide, however, can produce another very much rarer but much more serious side effect. This is a thickening of the tissues in the back of the abdominal wall. This can involve veins in the area and also put pressure on the ureters which are the narrow tubes which carry urine from the kidneys to the bladder. The condition is a low grade inflammation and is termed "retroperitoneal fibrosis". The patient who develops this complication may complain of a low backache. Swelling of one leg may be an early sign resulting from pressure from the thickened tissues on the veins carrying blood from the legs. In other patients a slight rise in temperature may occur and a diminished output in the daily amount of urine may be noticed.

As the toxic effects of methysergide do not usually occur until the drug has been used for several weeks, methysergide therapy is usually prescribed on an intermittent basis. If any side effects show themselves the drug is stopped immediately and any damage done is usually reversible. When a patient has been treated with the drug for a period of six months then therapy is interrupted for a period of at least six weeks.

Methysergide is made up in tablets containing two milligrams of the drug. The highest daily dose which can be taken is four tablets but fewer are advisable if satisfactory results can be obtained with less than a total of eight milligrams daily.

During an attack of migraine the branches of the external carotid artery become enlarged and distended. Work on methysergide has shown that it causes a very marked decrease in the blood flow of the external carotid artery circulation. Possibly methysergide is such an effective prophylactic therapy for migraine because it prevents the vascular dilation which is associated with the onset of pain in migraine.

Methysergide should not be used during pregnancy or by patients with kidney or heart disease. Its use has been largely superseded by the advent of newer drugs with fewer possible side effects.

Dixarit Therapy

This is a relatively new drug which was introduced into the treatment of migraine in Britain in 1969. Its major advantage is that it has no known harmful effects. In considering the use of any treatment with drugs one has to weigh the possible harmful effects of the drug against the benefits that one hopes will arise from it. When there is any doubt about it, it is best not to use the drug. One would not, for example, consider using methysergide for a patient with migraine unless the attacks were frequent and severe. Dixarit, like methysergide, is used as a preventive treatment. It appears to benefit about sixty to seventy per cent of patients. Although they may still suffer from headaches, these headaches become less frequent and less severe, and more amenable to analgesic therapy if they occur. The drug appears to be particularly helpful to patients who associate some of their attacks with the eating of certain foods such as chocolate, cheese, alcohol and citrus fruits. Some of these foods contain amines like tyramine and beta-phenylethylamine which have an effect on blood vessels and provoke a headache in a proportion of migraine sufferers. About one in three migraine subjects respond to dietary factors in this way. Dixarit acts by reducing the sensitivity or reactivity of blood vessels to any sort of stimuli and this is the basis on which it was introduced to migraine therapy.

It is of interest that Dixarit has also been found useful in treatment of the hot flushes that occasionally prove an embarassment to women during the menopause. This is hardly surprising when one considers that flushing is due to an overactivity of blood vessels.

Dixarit tablets contain twenty-five micrograms of clonidine hydrochloride. It has been found that clonidine in doses of one to two micrograms per kilogram of body weight decreases the response to peripheral blood vessels to any stimuli. This means that the blood vessels so treated do not dilate or constrict as much as normal. Dixarit tablets are bright blue. A starting dose is one tablet twice a day but the dosage can be gradually increased up to about six, or even in some patients to eight a day. The tablets should be spread as evenly as possible throughout the waking hours of the day. Larger doses than eight a day could have an effect on lowering the blood pressure.

The length of time for which a patient should stay on Dixarit treatment varies. Sometimes the dose has to be stepped up gradually until an effective level of anything up to eight tablets a day is reached. The maximum benefit from Dixarit is not always obtained before treatment has continued for up to three months and in doubtful cases it is well worthwhile continuing therapy for at least this length of time. Improvement is often dramatic and when it has been maintained for a few months it is worth tapering off Dixarit therapy gradually to see whether the improvement continues without the drug. Treatment can always be restarted again if needed.

Dixarit is a specific therapy for migraine which is not derived from the alkaloids of ergot. Patients taking Dixarit do not suffer from the side effects which make ergot a drug to be used with great caution.

Some patients on Dixarit complain of drowsiness. When this is severe it is worth trying the effect of two Dixarit tablets only a night. Dryness of the mouth occasionally occurs but usually passes off after two weeks. Dizziness, nausea and restlessness at night have also been reported. Skin rashes are a common manifestation of treatment with most drugs if toxic symptoms arise.

Dixarit should not be used in those who have a history of depressive illness. Occasionally Dixarit makes these symptoms worse. Depression in a migraine patient is difficult to judge. Anyone who suffered from constant, recurring thumping headaches might well get depressed. In such patients the relief which might accompany Dixarit therapy could well alter the sufferer's mental state.

The tragic thalidomide disaster has increased our awareness of the possible harmful effects of drugs on the unborn child. Extensive testing of pregnant animals has not shown Dixarit to have any harmful effects on the developing fetus. It is probably best, however, to avoid Dexarit during the first three months of pregnancy as this is the time when the developing fetus is most susceptible to harmful influences. In fact all but absolutely essential therapy would best be avoided at this time.

Migraine not uncommonly occurs in patients with a slightly raised blood pressure. These patients usually benefit from larger doses of the drug. Dixarit should not be used in migraine sufferers who are already receiving other treatment for a high blood pressure.

Pizotifen

This drug is marketed under the name of Sanomigran. It has much the same effect in migraine as methysergide but is unrelated to the latter and does not have the harmful possible side effects of methysergide. It can also be used in cluster headache. Like most drugs it should be avoided during pregnancy and in patients who have glaucoma, or suffer from urinary retention. The dose begins at 0.5 mg. three times daily and can be increased to a maximum of 6 mg a day. Occasionally patients on this drug put on weight or complain of drowsiness or fatigue.

Dihydroergotamine mesylate (DHE)

This drug is a semi synthetic ergot alkaloid which does not constrict blood vessels to the same extent as ergotamine itself. Because of the way in which they constrict blood vessels other ergotamine compounds cannot be used in prophylactic therapy and since it has a lesser but similar effect DHE should not be taken during pregnancy or by patients with vascular or heart disease. It has proved an effective prophylactic therapy in selected migraine sufferers. It is given in doses of 1.0 to 2.0 mg. three times a day.

A number of other drugs are used in the prophylactic therapy of migraine. Migraine is a disorder in which every patient has to be treated on an individual basis. There is no blanket therapy which will benefit all patients and the exact drugs prescribed by the doctor should be selected on a personal basis. Thus patients who have had frequent attacks of migraine, and who are not surprisingly depressed, sometimes improve on small doses of amitriptyline daily. This is an antidepressant drug but it also affects some of the changes in the blood thought to be associated with the onset of migraine attacks.

There are a number of drugs which alter the tone of blood vessels and also tend to reduce anxiety which have been introduced to migraine therapy.

Propanolol is in this category and is often particularly helpful in patients who also have a slightly raised blood pressure in addition to their headaches. Propanolol is usually used in doses of 40 mg two or three times a day.

Cyproheptadine is an antihistamine drug and also antagonises the actions of 5HT. Its value in migraine prophylaxis has not yet been fully assessed.

Anticonvulsant drugs

Diphenylhydantoin is sometimes used in the treatment of epilepsy and has occasionally been helpful in young migraine sufferers who have frequent attacks associated with minor changes on the electroencephalogram and a strong family history. Carbamazepine has been used in similar circumstances but neither of these drugs is a first choice in migraine prophylaxis.

Antihistamine drugs and diuretics have had their advocates from time to time, but are not drugs of choice.

Hormone therapy

Migraine reaches its peak incidence of over 10% in the female population between the ages of 20 and 45 years. This is undoubtedly related to the increased frequency of migraine at certain stages in the menstrual cycle. A chart recording the dates on which headaches occur and the times of menstruation over a length of time covering three months or more may prove very helpful. The normal menstrual cycle lasts twenty-eight days and where attacks occur most often at the time of ovulation or during or immediately after a menstrual perod it is probable that the symptoms are related to changes in the oestrogen level in the blood. These are times when the oestrogen levels are relatively high.

Occasionally patients are given treatment with oestrogens for such conditions as hot flushes. These patients sometimes report an increase in the severity of their headaches. Migrainous headaches occurring for the first time have also been reported in patients on oestrogen therapy.

A number of women notice that they seem to store water in their bodies before they develop an attack of migraine. The rings on their fingers, the waistbands of their skirts and their shoes may all feel tighter than usual. Oestrogen therapy sometimes produces water retention and the water retention which occurs naturally during certain phases of the menstrual cycle may reflect a rise in oestrogen levels in the body. This water retention is often noticed in the middle of the menstrual cycle or just before the onset of a menstrual period.

During the second half of the hormonal cycle when the incidence of headaches is less frequent, the hormone progesterone is being secreted. This has led to the use of progesterone as a treatment for women who suffer from migraine headaches bearing a clear relation to the menstrual cycle. The response to progesterone appears to be particularly good in those patients whose attacks occur just before or during menstruation. Hormonal therapy is occasionally helpful in women whose headaches occur in close association with the menstrual cycle or around the time of the menopause or after a hysterectomy. It is essential that hormone treatment is only taken under careful supervision.

Headaches on the "PILL"

Oral contraception should be avoided by women with a

strong family history of migraine and women using oral contraception should be given the pill with the lowest effective oestrogen content. Women who develop headaches for the first time, or whose headaches increase in severity when they are taking the "pill" should obtain expert advice at once.

TREATMENT OF AN ATTACK

Time is a factor of major importance when the symptoms of migraine begin to make themselves felt. Once the headache has really developed there is little the sufferer can do to ease it to any great degree. There are four main ways in which drugs can be given for migraine:

By mouth

By inhalation

In suppository form

By intramuscular injection

Experience at the Princess Margaret Migraine Clinic in London has shown that the best treatment of an acute attack of migraine is to lie down in a quiet room and take an anti-emetic, an analgesic and a tranquilizer.

Usually, however, the unfortunate victim has to struggle home from work or is unable to get to bed because the needs of small children cannot be ignored. Every migraine suffer knows the bliss of finally burying that pounding head in a pillow. No, rest in a darkened room may be the ideal solution, but circumstances are seldom ideal. So what does one do?

Analgesics

Aspirin remains the most commonly and effectively used therapy for a migraine attack. There are many analgesic tablets on the market containing such substances as aspirin, codeine, paracetamol and phenacetin. Thousands of tons of these analgesic tablets are consumed every year despite the fact that they are not without their harmful side effects. The main actions of aspirin are as an analgesic and an antipyretic. Recently it has been shown to have a marked action against prostaglandins. These are substances which are concerned in the production of inflammation and pain. The pain-relieving effect of aspirin increase with the dose of aspirin up to a maximum dose of 900 mg. Soluble or effervescent forms of aspirin should be used whenever possible because the absorption is quicker and the maximum levels of aspirin in the plasma of the blood are reached in about 45 minutes. Aspirin in large doses can cause nausea, vomiting, diarrhea, skin rashes, buzzing in the ears and giddiness. Aspirin also irritates the lining of the stomach and can occasionally produce ulceration and bleeding from the stomach. Phenacetin used to be a common ingredient in headache relieving powders and tablets. It is still found in some compounds, but should be avoided, as prolonged or excessive use can result in long lasting ill-effects particularly on the kidneys. Codeine is also contained in a number of compounds. It tends to have a constipating effect.

Paracetamol is commonly used and as it does not cause gastric irritation it may be preferred to aspirin. In large doses, over a prolonged period of time, however, it may cause liver damage. It is used in doses of 500 to 1000 mg.

All analgesic tablets should be taken with fluid to minimize their effect on the lining of the stomach. If you want to see what happens in your stomach when you take an aspirin tablet you can try keeping one between your gum and cheek while it dissolves. A raw inflamed area is likely to result. So even household remedies like aspirin should not be taken without due care. Furthermore prolonged and excessive use of analgesics can result in an almost continuous headache. Obviously if you feel a headache coming on you have got to take something to try to prevent it developing or to reduce its severity. The warning about analgesics is not intended to deter headache sufferers from taking them in moderation when absolutely necessary, but to draw attention to the fact that they can have harmful effects and should not be taken routinely like food.

Aspirin and other commonly used analgesics such as paracetamol and codeine are the treatment of choice in people who suffer from migraine. Phenacetin is best avoided in view of the kidney damage it is thought capable of causing.

Anti-Emetics

A high proportion of migraine sufferers, probably more than 90%, feel sick and often actually vomit during attacks. Gastric stasis also occurs which means that the stomach fails to contract effectively and this is probably a major reason why drugs taken by mouth are not adequately absorbed during an attack. Anti-emetics, particularly those that stimulate normal activity in the stomach and duodenum when gastrointestinal motility is reduced, not only diminish the symptoms of nausea and vomiting but increase the rate of absorption of drugs such as aspirin or paracetomol. An effective anti-emetic should therefore be taken 10 minutes before an analgesic is used.

Some migraine patients suffer from severe dizziness during an attack. This dizziness may in fact be the major symptom in a small proportion of patients. It can be treated with drugs used specifically for vertigo or dizziness.

Ergotamine tartrate

Ergot is obtained from the fungus *Claviceps purpurea.* This fungus is a parasite which grows on a number of grasses. Ergot, however, is usually obtained from rye. Ergot contains a number of alkaloids of which the most important are ergonovine, ergotoscine and ergotamine.

Ergot has no effect whatever when it is applied externally to the body. When it is given internally it has a powerful effect on the muscle of the pregnant uterus. For this reason ergot should never be prescribed for migraine during pregnancy.

It is nevertheless this action of ergot on the uterus which has provided its chief benefit to mankind in general and women in particular. An injection of an ergot compound is standard practice during the third stage of childbirth. During the first stage the uterus prepares to expel the child and the cervical canal through which the baby has to pass gradually dilates. At the end of the second stage the baby is born. It is attached to the mother by the umbilical cord which connects the baby to the placenta. This is a fleshy pad through which the developing embryo derives all its food and nourishment. The placenta is expelled during the third stage of labour leaving behind it a raw surface. The muscle of the uterus contracts to stop this raw area from bleeding excessively and this contraction is assisted very greatly by an injection of ergometrine maleate which is given intramuscularly during the third stage of labour. Ergot also has a direct action on blood vessels and causes them to constrict. It is this constricting action of ergot which sometimes results in peripheral gangrene in the limbs.

The ergot compound which is used most commonly in migraine is ergotamine. This was isolated from ergot in 1918. The blood vessels in the painful area of the head during a migraine attack are enlarged and painful and it is the constricting action of ergot which reduces the size of these vessels and relieves the pain.

Ergot can be given in four different ways, by mouth, by inhalation, by injection and in suppository form. If ergot is to be helpful it should be taken as soon as the patient feels that an attack is inevitable. If a patient is feeling sick and vomiting it is obviously useless taking ergotamine tablets by mouth. Some people cannot bear the thought of sticking a needle into themselves and they would obviously avoid ergot by injection. Suppositories provide the answer for a large number of sufferers but the route of administration chosen by an individual obviouly depends on various factors.

Ergotamine abuse is very common. Some migraine sufferers make an almost daily habit of using it. Despite warnings about the dangers of excessive ergot administration, these sufferers consider that they cannot do without it. They try to justify this by complaining that their headaches keep recurring without realising that the reason why they keep recurring is their constant use of ergotamine. Ergot abuse results in a vicious cycle of headaches. Prolonged ergot therapy can produce a paralysis of the nerves which supply the blood vessels and the latter stages in a migraine sufferer may be worse than the first. The headache becomes continuous.

Ergot can also produce other unwelcome side effects. The first symptoms of poisoning usually occur in the circulatory system. The sufferer may notice that his is always feeling chilly and cramps may cause trouble in the legs. A feeling of nausea may become marked and occasionally vomiting and diarrhea, which are common side effects of a large number of drugs, occur. Patients taking too much ergot sometimes notice tingling in their hands and feet. All these side effects provide a warning that should not be ignored and ergot therapy should be stopped at once if they occur.

Small doses of ergotamine are more effective in producing headache relief than large doses. The drug should be taken as early as possible in an attck.

Ergotamine tartrate is prepared in the following forms for the treatment of migraine.

Tablets. These are taken by mouth. A new tablet is available which does not have to be swallowed but can be held under the tongue until it dissolves. The dose of ergotamine tartrate contained in each tablet is one milligram. One tablet should be taken at the onset of the attack and this can be repeated in an hour if necessary. Not more than four tablets should be taken in twenty-four hours and not more than six tablets in a week.

Suppositories. Ergotamine suppositories contain two milligrams of ergotamine tartrate each. They often contain caffeine in addition as this is thought to enhance the effect of ergotamine. This is a particularly successful method of treating attacks in which the patient feels sick and is vomiting. One suppository should be used at the beginning of an attack and a further suppository can be used after an hour if needed. No more than three suppositories should be used in a day or five in a week. If a whole suppository is effective it is worth seeing whether a half will be effective in view of the benefits of decreasing the amount of ergot taken.

By Inhalation. Ergotamine can also be taken by inhalation. The Medihaler ergotamine contains 0.36 milligrams of ergotamine per puff or per inhalation. Migraine sufferers are advised to take one inhalation as soon as possible after the onset of an attack and to repeat this, if needed, at intervals of ten minutes for a maximum of five inhalations or puffs.

By Injection. Ergotamine tartrate injections contain 0.25 milligrams of ergotamine tartrate. They are given subcutaneously or intramuscularly. They can be repeated once only during an attack if necessary. No more than a maximum of four injections should be given during any one week.

There are a number of migraine sufferers who exceed the advisable limits of therapy with ergot. Very often these are the patients who have developed a cycle of incessant headaches as a result of ergot toxicity. These patients should seek the help of their doctors. A short spell in hospital is sometimes helpful to these sufferers while they are weaned on to less harmful treatment.

Treatment with ergot has been discussed at length. The reasons for this are obvious as it is a drug to which many migraine sufferers readily resort without always realizing fully its potential harm. Migraine sufferers should restrict their use of ergotamine-containing compounds to a minimum and be careful never to exceed the recommended dose.

Ergot should not be used during pregnancy, nor in prophylactic therapy and only extremely rarely in the treatment of children. At the Princess Margaret Migraine Clinic in London fewer than one in ten of the patients who are treated for acute attacks require ergotamine.

Dixarit Therapy

This is being tried in the treatment of an acute attack of migraine. Where a warning of an impending attack occurs in patients who are taking Dixarit as a prophylactic therapy it is often helpful to to take two extra tablets at once. Patients not on Dixarit therapy who feel that an attack is coming on should try to see whether or not the taking of one or two Dixarit tablets either averts the attack or reduces its usual severity. Dixarit appears to be a help to a number of migraine sufferers when it is taken in this way. In any case it is well worth giving it a trial in view of the lack of toxic effects.

Patients who are on prophylactic therapy with Dixarit often find that simple measures like aspirin are more effective than they used to be in alleviating their headaches when they occur.

REFERENCES

1. Domestic Medicine and Surgery, by J.H. Walsh, F.R.C.S. pub. Frederick Warne & Co., 1867.
2. One Dixarit tablet contains 0.025 mg clonidine hydrochloride.

HEADACHE AND CHEMISTRY

The father of modern chemistry, Antoine Laurent Lavoisier, died on the guillotine. Born in Paris in 1743, he became farmer general of taxes in 1768. He did this in order to obtain the means to pursue his chemical investigations but it was his role as farmer general of taxes that led to his death in 1794 during the French revolution. About 20 years earlier a Swedish chemist Carl Scheele, and an English man, Joseph Priestly, had both discovered oxygen independently. It was Lavoisier, however, who recognized oxygen as a chemical element and showed quantitatively the similarity between chemical oxidation and the process of respiration.

Priestly began studying chemistry while he was a presbyterian minister in Leeds. His religious writings caused great controversy and when his home was destroyed by mob violence he moved to America. In 1794 he settled down in Northumberland, Pa. and died in 1804.

A hundred years earlier Robert Boyle, a philosopher and alchemist, was questioning the basis of the chemical theory of his day. The alchemists searched not only for ways of turning baser metals into gold but also for an elixir of life. Their studies of nature were linked with astrology and mysticism and they sensed vaguely that a knowledge of the chemical transformation of matter might lead to power to benefit man. Their investigations were combined with the search for the philosopher's stone. This substance was supposed to possess wonderful properties that could turn lead into gold, cure disease, restore youth and prolong life. Methods have changed but the pursuits of the alchemists were not so far removed from those of many a modern man although we frequently wrap our philosopher's stone in a gaudier, commercial package. The alchemists tried to discover the substance of life and although this approach was necessary largely philosophical they were nevertheless the forerunners of modern science. In the sixteenth century the iatrochemists taught that the main purpose of the study of matter was to make medicines and aid the physician.

Boyle lived from 1627 to 1691. He taught that the proper object of chemistry was to determine the composition of substances. His contemporary, John Mayow, observed the fundamental analogy between the process of animal respiration, whereby oxygen is taken into the body with the breakdown of carbohydrate and release of energy, and the burning of organic matter in air.

Photosynthesis in plants was another biological process which attracted the attention of chemists in the late eighteenth century, and the combined work of Joseph Priestly, Jan Ingenhousz and Jean Senebier showed that this is essentially the reverse of respiration. In respiration oxygen is taken into the body and with the breakdown of carbohydrate energy is released and water and carbon dioxide are formed. In photosynthesis in plants the reverse process occurs. Water and carbon dioxide are taken into the plant and, in the presence of chlorophyll, carbohydrate is formed. The simple equations for the two processes are shown as follows:

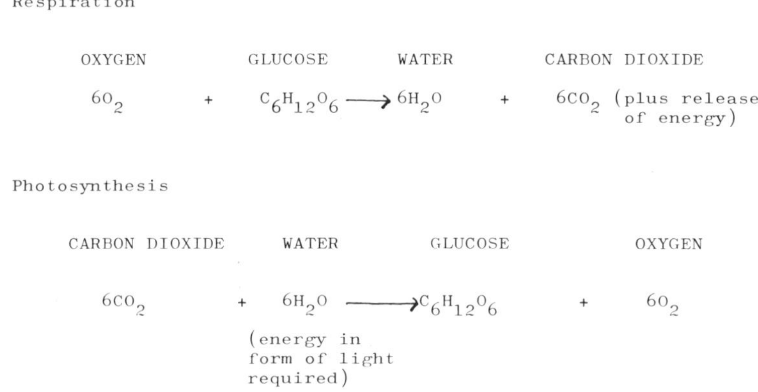

Despite these early observations on living matter progress in biochemistry was dependent on the development of structural organic chemistry which did not occur until the nineteenth century. Obviously the molecular composition of a substance had to be known before it could be synthesized.

Progress was impeded by the Vitalists who took the view that organic matter could not be synthesized. When Friedrich Woehler achieved the laboratory synthesis of urea the Vitalists countered this blow to their theory by taking refuge in the fact that urea is a breakdown product in the body, and not a product of synthesis. The ensuing success of organic chemists in synthesizing many organic compounds forced the Vitalists to retreat. It is axiomatic in modern biochemistry that the chemical laws which apply to inanimate materials are equally applicable to the living cell and can completely describe the living cell.

In the nineteenth century two men in particular were responsible for developing the application of chemical methods to living matter. Justus von Liebig was born in 1803 in Germany. At that time it was difficult to advance in chemistry in Germany as there was a dearth of laboratories for the practical training of students and the subject was taught largely from textbooks. Liebig went to study in Paris and then returned to Giessen where he found the first great teaching and research laboratory applying chemical methods to living processes. Liebig studied the great chemical cycle in nature and pointed out that this cycle is maintained by a continuous process of animal decay and plant synthesis. The application of this work to agricultural science became clear and led to the use of fertilizers for the soil. It is interesting that Liebig was the first person to synthesize chloroform.

In France at the same time Louis Pasteur was founding the science of bacteriology. Throughout his life he was extremely industrious and even on his death-bed he exhorted his pupils to work. Pasteur showed that living organisms are responsible for the process of fermentation, putrefaction and disease. His name remains with us as a household word. The pasteurization of milk evolved from his demonstration of the fact that treatment of liquids with mild heat for a certain period of time destroys microorganisms which might otherwise cause disease. Among some other results of his work were the introduction of a vaccine to be used against smallpox and the method of preventive innoculation against rabies. It was Pasteur's work in bacteriology which enabled Lister in Britain to introduce antiseptic techniques into the practice of surgery.

Another great scientist of that day was the Frenchman Claude Bernard. Having failed in his ambitions for a literary career he trained as a physician. He brought a new approach to the problems of disease and recognized the importance of applying chemistry to medicine. He discovered glycogen and the fact that it is stored in the liver. Glycogen is the form in which glucose is stored in the body.

Gradually the need to link chemistry with physiology became apparent and a new branch of science was recognized. The term biochemistry was introduced in 1900. As the ultimate goal of biochemistry is to achieve a complete understanding of the processes of life within the cell and at a molecular level, it is obvious that as far as one can see into the future every step forward in biochemical knowledge will lead to endless new avenues of interest demanding exploration. Every disorder of functions in the body must result in biochemical changes which differ from the normal pattern. It is not unreasonable to suppose that even those disorders whose aetiology remains obscure at present will eventually yield their secrets to the curiosity, probing and skill of the biochemist.

In 1838 a Dutch biochemist called Mulder named a substance recently isolated from living tissue "protein". The word protein was derived from the Greek meaning "holding first place". It was an appropriate name as proteins are essential to life. Proteins are formed from chains of amino-acids which link together into polypeptide chains. About twenty different aminoacids occur in nature, eight of which are essential constituents of the diet in so far as the human organism is unable to synthesize them itself. Each protein molecule is likely to contain all twenty aminoacids arranged in a variety of sequences. It is the sequence of different aminoacids which gives individual proteins their specific properties. Enzymes form a particularly important group of proteins as they are produced by living cells and act as catalysts in the chemical reactions upon which life depends. Each different enzyme in the body controls only one particular action, and thus the working of an individual cell depends on the kind of enzymes it contains.

Digestion is the process by which the molecules in the food we eat are broken down into smaller molecules which are then absorbed into the body and built up into the material that composes our own tissues. Our food consists of three major constituents, carbohydrate, protein and fat. The vitamins and minerals essential to health are also contained in a balanced diet. The body forms different enzymes for the purpose of breaking down the food we eat. There are starch splitting enzymes, fat splitting enzymes and protein splitting enzymes.

The body continually requires and uses up energy. It obtains this energy by combining the carbon and hydrogen of the food we eat with the oxygen we breathe. The main energy requirements of the body are obtained from the breakdown of glucose which is obtained from the digestion of carbohydrates in the diet. Under normal conditions a constant amount of glucose is kept available in the bloodstream for immediate use by the body cells. Glucose is also stored in the form of glycogen, chiefly in the liver and also in muscle. This reserve can be mobilized if necessary. If an excess of glucose remains available when the body stores are adequately filled, then the liver cells convert surplus glucose into fat. The fat stores provide a further insurance against need and can be called upon if the glycogen stores should become depleted. This could arise, for example, during prolonged starvation. Fat, however, is a less efficient source of energy than glucose, and the breakdown of fat results in the production of certain substances called ketone bodies. These are poisonous to the body and produce a characteristic smell in the patient like pear drops. This smell is sometimes very noticeable in children who have been starved and who are breaking down their body fat to provide energy. Similarly untreated diabetic patients become ketotic as, despite the fact that their blood may be loaded with sugar, they are unable to use it. Their bodies have to resort to the breakdown of fat to supply energy.

Proteins are only called upon to supply energy as a last resort. This means that the body has reached the stage of breaking down its own tissues in its attempt to survive. Protein is an essential constituent of the diet and eight amino-acids are vital to life. The body is unable to make these eight amino-acids which are found in foods such as meat, dairy products and some vegetables. The essential amino-acids are

Lysine	Valine
Leucine	Methionine
Isoleucine	Phenylalanine
Threonine	Tryptophan

The reason why we are interested in these essential amino acids is that when they are metabolised in the body some of them produce amines which are capable of affecting the size of blood vessels. These amines are called vasoactive amines. Tryptophan is important because it produces the vasoactive amine 5-hydroxytryptamine. An amine is formed when carbon dioxide is removed from an amino acid. The general formula for this is as follows:

$$R.CH.NH_2COOH \rightarrow R.CH_2\,NH_1$$

$$\text{Amino Acid} \rightarrow \text{minus } CO_2 \rightarrow \text{Amine}$$

Amines can also be obtained from ammonia. The formula for ammonia is NH_3 and an amine is formed when one or more of the hydrogen atoms in ammonia is replaced by other radicals. Because there are three hydrogen atoms in ammonia it is possible to obtain primary, secondary and tertiary amines depending on whether one, two or three hydrogen atoms have been replaced.

The chief vasoactive amines implicated in headaches are: Adrenaline, noradrenaline, dopamine, octopamine, histamine, tyramine, β-phenylethylamine and 5-hydroxytryptamine.

When we think about the biochemistry of headache we are considering headaches which result from vascular changes occurring in response to the presence of increased levels of vasoactive amines in the blood. Thus the type of headache with which we are chiefly concerned in this category is migraine.

PLATELETS AND 5-HYDROXYTRYPTAMINE (5HT)

A number of vasoactive amines appear to be concerned in producing an attack of migraine. They include adrenaline, noradrenaline, tyramine and 5-hydroxytryptamine. The most common cause of migraine is stress. We know that the blood levels of adrenaline and noradrenaline rise during stress. Tyramine is a constituent of some of the foods that have been cited as precipitants of some attacks. Other vaso active amines in food that are probably linked with occasional migraine attacks are octopamine and β-phenylethylamine. These are mentioned in more detail in the section on headaches and food. There is one vasoactive amine which appears to play a major role in migraine. This is 5-hydroxytryptamine which is often abbreviated to 5HT and sometimes also called serotonin.

5HT was first isolated from blood in 1948. It is contained in small coin shaped particles in the blood called platelets. Blood has 200,000 to 400,000 platelets per cubic millimeter. The chief function of the platelets is in connection with blood clotting. If there is a break in the wall of a blood vessel the platelets clump together to form a clot which plugs the breach and stops the bleeding.

A substance called ADP (adenosine diphosphate) is present in platelets and is responsible for their clotting powers. When bleeding occurs platelets adhere to the damaged site of the vessels. They release ADP which causes more platelets to collect at the site of injury. They also discharge 5-hydroxytryptamine (5HT) which causes the blood vessels in the area to constrict and thereby reduces further bleeding.

Platelets clump together or aggregate in response to a number of different factors. We have already mentioned ADP. Among other factors causing platelet aggregation are adrenaline, noradrenaline, tyramine, and 5HT itself.

It is possible to employ methods to compare the rate and degree of platelet aggregation in different samples of blood plasma. Plasma is blood from which all blood cells have been removed. If plasma is enriched with platelets and ADP is added to it then the rate at which the platelets aggregate can be measured. Similarly various substances can be added to such platelet enriched plasma in order to see whether and how they affect the rate of aggregation of the platelets. The aggregation of platelets is a subject of interest in migraine because it has been shown that, whether or not they have a headache when the blood sample is taken and whether or not they are on drug therapy, the platelets of migraine sufferers show an increased tendency to aggregate.

Furthermore during a migraine attack a so-called "releasing factor" is present in the plasma of a migraine subject which causes the platelets to release 5HT. The presence of this releasing factor has been demonstrated by experiments in which plasma obtained from migraine subjects during an attack has been shown to release 5HT from platelets obtained from the same subjects during a headache free period.

The platelets of migraine subjects have been shown to release their 5HT more readily in response to tyramine than the platelets of control subjects.

Levels of 5HT in the blood bear a definite relation to the onset of migraine in migraine sufferers. Although there is no difference between the 5HT levels of normal and migrainous subjects between attacks, it has been shown that in the prodromal phase of migraine, that is just prior to the onset of headache, 5HT levels in the blood sometimes rise to three times their normal levels. They fall to a statistically significant degree during the headache phase. Despite the fact taht the level falls at the time when the headache is most severe, the level in the migraine sufferer may still be above the levels in normal control subjects at this time. When investigating changes in the levels of 5HT it is essential to compare levels in the same individual all the time and not to try to compare them in different individuals.

When substances undergo changes in the body their end products or metabolites are often excreted in the urine. The major metabolite of 5HT is 5-hydroxyindoleacetic acid (5HIAA). The amounts of this substance found in the urine are often increased in a migraine attack. Changes in amount may occur over a very limited period only and frequent collections of urine may be necessary over a period of twenty-four hours to make sure that any change in amount is detected.

5HT has several actions. It constricts large arteries and veins and dilates smaller arteries or arterioles in the limbs of man. It also prevents the excretion of water from the body and stimulates the activity of the intestine. These last two effects are interesting as some migraine sufferers complain of water retention before an attack begins and the onset of migraine is occasionally accompanied by diarrhea. Whether or not these symptoms are due to the rise in level of 5-hydroxytryptamine, or even associated with this at all is not yet clear. During a migraine attack the level of 5HT in the blood falls and if it is then given intravenously the symptoms of headache are often relieved. The headache is often also relieved when the sufferer vomits and it is interesting to note that vomiting causes 5HT levels to rise in the body. Possibly the relief of headache following vomiting is associated with this. The side effects of 5HT are restlessness, nausea, faintness and flushing.

In carrying out research into migraine various methods have been used in attempts to induce an attack. Reserpine is a drug that has sometimes been employed for this purpose. Reserpine acts by liberating vasoactive amines including 5HT from nerve endings. Amine stores appear to be particularly sensitive to releasing stimuli in migraine subjects. The ability of reserpine to release amines declines with increasing age in patients. Possibly this has something to do with the fact that the incidence of migraine also falls with increasing age. Significant rises in the urinary excretion of 5HIAA have been shown to occur after reserpine-induced migraine.

Indirect confirmatory evidence that 5HT plays an important role in migraine is provided by the fact that one of the most successful prophylactic therapies in migraine is the use of methysergide. This drug acts as a 5HT antagonist.

MONO-AMINE OXIDASE AND TYRAMINE

Enzymes are protein substances which are present in exceedingly small amounts in the body. Despite this fact they are of vital importance. Enzymes are substances which, without themselves undergoing any change, cause other substances to change. They act as catalysts in chemical reactions, that is they speed up reactions in the body.

When we think about migraine we are interested in a group of enzymes called the monoamine oxidase enzymes. They are concerned in the breakdown in the body of the vasoactive amines that have been mentioned. The monoamine oxidase enzymes add oxygen and remove ammonia from amines according to the general formula.

$$RCH_2NH_2 + O_2 + H_2O \rightarrow RCHO + NH_3 + H_2O_2$$

Ammonia is formed in this process and it is interesting to note that when a small group of migraine sufferers with classical migraine were investigated their blood levels of ammonia were found to be raised.

Monoamine oxidase enzymes are widespread in the

body. Their concentration differs in various sites. For example, they are present in relatively large amounts in the liver, salivary glands, kidney and digestive tract. They are found in fairly large amounts in the adrenal glands, the uterus, the pancreas, the lungs, spleen and brain. They are absent or present only in very low quantities in heart muscle, red blood cells and plasma.

In 1952 a new group of drugs was introduced into the treatment of tuberculosis. These drugs acted as inhibitors of monoamine oxidase enzymes in the body; and it was observed that some of the tuberculous patients who were treated in this way became noticeably more cheerful. Because of this rise in spirits the drug was tried in patients suffering from depression and a marked improvement in some of them was soon apparent. This led to the introduction of monoamine oxidase inhibitor drugs on a large scale for the treatment of depression.

Despite the fact that thousands of patients in the United States were treated with these drugs no adverse reactions to them were reported for three years. Then reports gradually filtered in of severe headaches associated with a rise in blood pressure which occurred in some of the patients on this therapy. Careful detective work established that these headaches were associated with the eating of certain foods, notably cheese. The substance contained in the cheese that was responsible for those reactions was found to be a substance called tyramine, a name derived from the Greek word for cheese. Tyramine is a vasoactive monoamine.

It is normally broken down in the body by the action of monoamine oxidase and exerts an action on blood vessels both directly and through releasing noradrenaline from its stores.

Although cheese was the main food to be incriminated in the headache reactions occurring in patients on monoamine oxidase inhibitor drugs certain other foods were also found to have similar harmful effects. These foods also were subsequently found to contain vasoactive amines. Owing to the inhibition of monoamine oxidase by the monoamine oxidase inhibitor therapy which the patients were receiving, the vasoactive amines in the various foods were not broken down and rendered harmless as they would normally have been and the headache reactions resulted.

Since that time any patients who are treated with monoamine oxidase inhibitor drugs are warned against eating certain foods. The list includes

Cheese	Chocolate
Marmite	Broad beans
Yoghurt	Alcoholic beverages
Pickled herring	

The fascinating fact is that the foods which patients on monoamine oxidase inhibitor drugs are advised to avoid eating are very similar to the foods which have been repeatedly incriminated over many years as migraine precipitants. Thus alcohol, cheese, fish, beans, dairy produce and chocolate have all been cited as precipitants of migraine attacks in migraine sufferers who link some of their headaches with food factors.

Fortunately the reason for the headache and high blood pressure reactions which occurred in patients on the monoamine oxidase inhibitors when they ate cheese was soon identified as the presence of the vasoactive amine tyramine in the cheese.

The next question was obvious. Would tyramine in any way affect migraine sufferers who linked some of their attacks with the eating of the same foods that caused headaches in patients on the monoamine oxidase inhibitor drugs? In particular, could tyramine taken in pure form by mouth precipitate a headache in this group of migraine sufferers?

As this is the area of research in which I have been working perhaps you will forgive me for writing about it in a personal way. To begin with I would like to say how grateful I shall always be to Dr. Marcia Wilkinson for letting me work in her Migraine Clinic when I first wanted to investigate this aspect of migraine, and to the Wellcome Trustees who have kindly supported this work.

Patients who were attending the migraine clinic at the Elizabeth Garrett Anderson Hospital were questioned about dietary factors in relation to their headaches. Those who gave a clearcut history of an association between certain articles of food and their headaches were carefully selected and asked whether they would be willing to take part in an investigation. They were told that capsules containing food extracts would be sent to them by post. As patients are unlikely to develop a migraine attack again within forty-eight hours of having a headache they were advised not to test any capsule less than forty-eight hours after an attack. They were also warned against testing a capsule when they thought a headache might be due. For instance if a patient usually had an attack of migraine every two weeks it would clearly be pointless testing a capsule twelve days after the last attack.

Two sets of capsules were prepared. They looked identical but one set contained tyramine and the other lactose. Lactose is a completely innocuous substance which is often used in investigations of this nature as it cannot possibly exert any effect of any sort.

Within a few weeks it became clear that oral tyramine could precipitate an attack of migraine within 24 hours in a significant proportion of migraine patients.

The results of a number of administrations of 100 mg. of tyramine and identical looking capsules containing lactose in 50 patients with dietary migraine:

Substance	No effect	Migraine attack
Lactose	60	6
Tyramine	20	80

The testing of tyramine to see whether or not it might precipitate an attack of migraine was only a beginning. Tyramine acts directly on blood vessels. It also releases noradrenaline, another vasoactive amine, from its stores in the body and noradrenaline has a powerful action in blood vessels.

Tyramine is broken down in the body by two main methods. One route is through the action of the enzyme monoamine oxidase. The other way in which tyramine is metabolized in the body is by linkage with a sulphate radicle to form tyramine sulphate. In addition to these two disposal routes a certain amount of tyramine is excreted in a free form in urine.

You may be wondering what effect, if any, large doses of tyramine by mouth have on people who do not suffer from migraine. This was subsequently investigated in three hundred volunteers. Tyramine was found to have no effect whatever in people who never get a headache. In people who occasionally suffer from headaches it sometimes produced a headache which varied according to the usual headache pattern.

The fact that tyramine appeared to be exerting an abnormal effect in the selected migraine suffers made me wonder whether or not migraine sufferers had a defect in their monoamine oxidase enzyme system. This would go some way towards explaining why they got headaches when they ate tyramine-containing foods, in a similar way to that in which headaches occurred in patients whose enzyme symptom was depressed by monoamine oxidase inhibitor drugs.

So the next step in this biochemical detective story was to estimate the monoamine oxidase levels in a group of migraine patients and in a group of non-migrainous control subjects. Monoamine oxidase levels in the blood platelets of both groups were estimated. Anyone who enjoys hunting for clues and piecing them together will appreciate the excitement when significantly less of the enzyme was found in the platelets of the migraine sufferers than in the control group.

Subsequently monoamine oxidase levels were measured in migraine patients during headache attacks, and the platelet enzyme content found to be even more markedly reduced.

MIGRAINE HYPOTHESIS

There is a story about a group of men who were given limited space and time in a pitch dark room and told to examine a very large elephant. They were then asked to describe what they had found. One man who had caught hold of the trunk, described a long tubular snake-like creature. Another, who had felt a leg, described an animal like the bark of a tree. Yet a third had examined an ear and described a flat, flabby fish-like object. Any hypothesis for a disorder is like an attempt to describe the whole of the elephant. In putting forward my hypothesis for migraine I am saying that the whole of the elephant of migraine is a platelet abnormality. This abnormality of platelet function may be inherited in patients who give a strong family history of migraine or acquired, as in the case of previously headache-free women who develop migraine attacks when they begin using oral contraceptives.

In suggesting that a platelet abnormality is the primary cause of migraine I am placing migraine into an entirely new category, among the most common disorders of the blood.

Platelets are small, irregularly shaped discs, numbering from 200,000 to 400,000 per cubic ml. of blood. They are roughly one half to one third the size of red cells but possess no iron containing pigment like the haemoglobin of red cells. Platelets also differ from cells as they have no nuclei.

The way in which platelets behave is influenced by a number of factors. These include genetic factors, sex, age, and the effects of certain drugs, hormones and antigens. Most of these factors are also relevant to the incidence of migraine. In particular the genetic control of platelet behavior could explain the commonly observed familial incidence of migraine. When questioned in an out-patient clinic roughly six out of every ten migraine sufferers give a strong family history of the disorder.

Any hypothesis for a disorder has to satisfy a number of criteria. It has to explain the symptoms of the disorder as well as to fit in with the biochemical and pathological findings. It also has to explain why a particular line of treatment is helpful.

We define migraine as a headache, usually affecting chiefly one side of the heat, which recurs at intervals. It is often associated with nausea and vomiting. Migraine has been classified into two groups, common migraine and classical migraine. Common migraine is about twice as frequent as classical migraine. In classical migraine the symptoms of unilateral headache, nausea and vomiting are preceded by preomonitory signs called an aura. These signs are a warning and herald an attack. They are usually followed by the onset of headache within a period of approximately fifteen minutes. The signs are usually visual and they vary from one patient to another although they remain fairly constant to the individual person.

It is in classical migraine that the effects of abnormal platelet behavior are most clearly seen.

The most common precipitant of migraine is stress. Stress in this context includes such states as anxiety, excitement, fatigue, anger, or exertion. Hormonal changes appear to play a role in some women and probably account for the fact that the incidence of migraine rises from the figure of

8% in the general population to nearly 20% in women between the ages of 20 and 45 years. The increased incidence of migraine in some women on the pill is also linked with hormonal factors. Roughly one in three migraine sufferers report that dietary factors are associated with some of their attacks, chocolate, cheese and alcohol being the most commonly cited food precipitants. A small proportion of sufferers report that a lack of food can cause an attack. The important clinical observation on the causes of migraine is that they are cumulative in effect.

All of the causes of migraine are associated with changes in vaso active amine metabolism. The amines concerned are:

> Noradrenaline
> Adrenaline
> 5-hydroxytryptamine (5HT)
> Tyramine
> β-phenylethylamine (BPEA)

There appears to be a threshold level which varies from one sufferer to the next, but when the trigger is sufficiently powerful and the threshold is exceeded, an attack follows.

All the amines listed are dealt with in the body, at least in part, by the mono-amine oxidase group of enzymes (MAO). Platelets contain mono amine oxidase. MAO activity in platelets has been found to be reduced in migraine sufferers and falls significantly during attacks. MAO activity also increases with age which may contribute to the lessening of migraine attacks with increasing age. In women, a peak in MAO activity has been reported at the middle of the menstrual cycle with a nadir 5 to 11 days later. This may be linked with the high incidence of migraine attacks in some women just before menstruation.

The role of 5HT in migraine has been extensively studied. It has been shown that 5HT levels rise before the onset of headache and fall sharply during the headache phase. The chief breakdown product of 5HT in the body is 5-hydroxyindole acetic acid (5HIAA) which is excreted in the urine. The excretion of 5HIAA is increased during migraine attacks.

The total amount of 5HT in the blood is contained in the platelets. Platelets release their 5HT when they clump together. This clumping is called platelet aggregation. The platelets of migraine sufferers have been shown to aggregate more readily than those of control subjects.

The common factors causing platelet aggregation are
  Adenosine diphosphate (ADP)
  5-Hydroxytryptamine (5HT)
  Adrenaline
  Noradrenaline
  Thrombin
  Collagen
  Arachidonic Acid (AA)
There is a close link between these factors and the causes of migraine. Adrenaline, noradrenaline and arachidonic acid levels rise with stress which is the chief cause of migraine. Thrombin and collagen levels in blood are affected by hormonal factors.

Migraine precipitating foods contain vasoactive amines, notably tyramine and β-phenylethylamine. Both of these amines release noradrenaline from nerve terminals in the body. In addition tyramine has been shown to release 5HT from platelets. The platelets of migraine subjects out of an attack are more sensitive to the tyramine releasing effect than platelets from control subjects.

While the causes of migraine are clearly linked with factors causing platelet aggregation there is just as striking a link between the drugs used in the treatment of migraine and drugs that inhibit platelet aggregation. Aspirin, methysergide and dihydroergotamine are examples of these drugs.

In the prodromal phase of migraine a proportion of sufferers experience symptoms similar to the symptoms of transient cerebral ischaemia which arise in a much older age group of patients with hardening of their cerebral arteries. These effects of cerebral ischaemia are reversible within a period of 10 to 15 minutes. The aura of migraine occurs within this period of time. If abnormal platelet behavior resulting in platelet aggregation and 5HT release is the chief cause of migraine then the prodromal symptoms could arise from ischaemic episodes resulting from the temporary blockage of small cerebral vessels by platelet aggregates. Not only would this reduce the blood flow in the vessels but the release of 5HT which accompanies aggregation, in the presence of diminished mono amine oxidase enzyme levels would cause vasoconstriction and enhance the ischaemic effect.

The area of the brain dealing with vision has been found to be particularly sensitive to the effects of even very minor reductions in blood supply. This may account for the frequency of visual symptoms during the prodromal phases of migraine. A generalised abnormality of blood flow in small blood vessels in migraine subjects has been observed. Conjunctival, lip, tongue and nail fold vessels were examined microscopically in migraine sufferers during and between attacks and showed an increase in red cell aggregation. This suggests that in migraine sufferers there may be some slowing in the blood flow through small vessels which becomes more marked during an attack.

If we accept that platelet aggregation and 5HT release are responsible for the ischaemia producing the prodromal symptoms of migraine then we are left with the headache to explain.

Cerebral blood flow studies in the baboon have shown that an infusion of 5HT into the external carotid artery increases its blood flow by several hundred per cent. This is opposite to its effect in the internal carotid supply where the flow is decreased. Some of the branches of the external carotid artery pass into the skull and dilation of these vessels could produce the meningeal type of pain which is characteristic of severe migraine. The middle meningeal artery is a branch of the first part of the maxillary artery which is the larger terminal branch of the external carotid artery. Having entered the skull through the foramen spinosum its branches extend over the temporal and parietal area of the skull and into the orbit. These are the most common sites of pain in migraine.

5HT is known to be closely concerned with pain production. Studies of microvascular injury have shown that once a tissue has been inflamed it carries a memory of the event. This imprinting has an important influence on the nervous system and may explain why pain in a migraine attack is often experienced in the same site by the individual sufferer.

We know that plasma 5HT levels rise prior to the onset of headache in migraine and fall sharply during the headache phase. There have been reports of migraine occurring for the first time in patients who had an illness in which sudden falls occurred in the numbers of their platelets. The headaches in these patients occurred in conjunction with the rapid destruction of platelets, in fact when a sudden release of 5HT was followed by a dramatic fall. A rapid rise followed by a fall in 5HT levels appears to be a vital factor in migraine. This change could well be masked when 5HT levels at different stages are compared in groups of patients and not in individuals during a single attack.

If we accept that this hypothesis would explain familial miraine we still have to account for migraine attacks arising for the first time later in life, and for the isolated attack. The occurrence of migraine has been noted in a proportion of women using oral contraception. This can be explained by the effect of oral contraceptives on platelets.

Classical migraine has been reported as occurring for the first time in healthy young boxers and footballers following blows on the head. Any unitary theory of causation of attacks of migraine must account for the prodromal symptoms, which included incapacitating visual field defects, and occurred immediately after the injury.

Both trauma and exertion are linked with an increase in platelet aggregation. In the extreme circumstances cited this may have been sufficient to initiate the chain of events described.

A similar explanation probably applies to a young man who had two episodes of transient neurological symptoms following extreme exercise and the ingestion of cheese and chocolate. In addition to the effects of exercise the vasoactive amines contained in cheese and chocolate could also have had a platelet aggregating effect and the tyramine content of cheese might well have had an additive effect in causing 5HT release.

Although in the extreme circumstances described platelet aggregation may have been the chief factor in precipitating the symptoms of a migraine attack, an increase in platelet aggregation alone is unlikely to explain the pathogenesis of migraine as a whole. Increased platelet aggregation is found in other conditions, such as diabetes, and no association with migraine headaches has been found in diabetic patients. Nor has a low level of platelet 5HT, such as that reported in mongolism, been linked with headache. Headaches have, however, been reported in patients with lowered mono-amine oxidase levels in the blood, secondary to mono-amine oxidase inhibitor therapy (MAOI) and in association with the ingestion of tyramine containing foods. Tyramine releases 5HT from platelets and the headaches reported in the patients on mono-amine inhibitor therapy may have been associated with a sudden release of 5HT following the ingestion of tyramine. The platelets of migraine subjects have been shown to be more sensitive to the tyramine releasing effect than platelets from control subjects. The presence of mono-amine oxidase has been demonstrated in the walls of blood vessels and cyclical variations during the menstrual cycle in mono-amine oxidase levels in the lining of the uterus have been reported. It is feasible that variations in arterial mono-amine oxidase also occur, and that this is an additive factor in the action of 5HT on cerebral vessels.

It appears that a number of conditions have to be met before an attack of migraine occurs. The various factors operating to produce these conditions will vary from one individual to another but the end result will be an increase in platelet aggregation, a rise in plasma 5HT followed by a fall and a diminution in platelet mono-amine oxidase. Some of these conditions are present individually in other disorders. An increase in platelet aggregation alone is not enough to precipitate migraine except possibly under extreme circumstances such as the stress, trauma and exertion associated with the rarely reported incidence of migraine attacks occurring in isolation in footballers during a match or boxers during a fight. A fall in platelet MAO alone is not enough. Headaches only occurred in patients on MAOI therapy when they ate tyramine-containing foods.

In conclusion, a number of conditions combine in migraine subjects, each of which is closely linked with platelet function and can explain the sequence of biochemical events leading to an attack of migraine. These are a diminution in platelet mono-amine oxidase, an increase in platelet aggregation and a rise in 5HT followed by a fall. The diversity of symptoms arising in migraine becomes explicable when we consider that the factors operating to produce an attack are so variable and that the degree, site and extent of platelet aggregation will differ from one patient to another. Thus my hypothesis postulates that abnormal platelet function is not only a major factor in the pathogenesis of migraine attacks but their prime cause.

MIGRAINE AND EPILEPSY

This section on migraine and epilepsy will start with some figures about the frequency with which these disorders occur. There appears to be a shadowy relationship between them but the way in which they might be linked, if indeed they are, is still very vague. Migraine is about ten times more common than epilepsy. Epilepsy occurs in about one in every two hundred members of the general population. It is thought to occur two to six times more often in people who suffer from migraine than in other people. The figures given for the incidence of migraine in the population vary between five and ten people in a hundred. Epilepsy, like migraine, sometimes runs in families and when they are asked about it a third of the sufferers from epilepsy state that other members of their families suffer or have suffered from epilepsy. Interestingly enough, migraine also seems to occur somewhat more frequently in the families of sufferers from epilepsy than in the rest of the population. One in four epileptics give a family history of migraine.

There are other points on which migraine and epilepsy share similarities. Both conditions are episodic and recur at intervals. In the intervening periods, which may vary from days to months, the sufferers may be completely fit. Patients who suffer from migraine sometimes have a warning that an attack is likely to occur. Disturbances of vision may occur and the sufferer may see zigzag lights called fortification spectra. On rarer occasions a migraine sufferer may complain of loss of feeling in a limb. Similar aura or premonitary signs can also occur before an attack of epilepsy. An epileptic fit is characterized by a brief loss of consciousness. On rare occasions migraine sufferers have been known to lose consciousness during an attack. Epilepsy and migraine can both occur in the same patient and it is not unreasonable to suggest that there is some common basis in the reasons for which they both occur.

The fact that electrical activity occurs in nerves was discovered by an Italian physiologist, Luigi Galvani. He was born in Bologna in 1737 and gained his reputation as an anatomist. While doing some experiments on frogs he noticed that twitching of the muscles occurred when simultaneous contact took place between the muscle and two different metals, iron and copper. Galvani then conducted an experiment in which he placed one metal on the muscle of the frog and a different metal on the nerve to the muscle. In this way an electric current was produced and the muscle twitched. Galvani enunciated his theory of animal electricity in 1791. He died in 1798.

Electrical activity is going on all the time in the nerve cells. The fact that the brain shows electrical activity was first demonstrated in 1875. At that time some experimental work was done on animals. By attaching electrodes to the surface of the brain, and using a very sensitive galvanometer, shifts of between three and five millivolts could be measured. A recording made directly from the brain surface is called an electro-corticogram. For very obvious reasons this sort of investigation cannot be done in ordinary circumstances but the technique of electroencephalography in man has evolved from it.

An electroencephalogram (EEG) is the record obtained when electrodes are placed on the scalp. Small silver discs are used as electrodes. This investigation has some similarity with the very common technique of electrocardiography (ECG), which is used to obtain tracings of the electrical activity of the heart. When an electrocardiogram is taken the record obtained from the patient who is being investigated is compared with a record typical of a normal heart. It is then possible to see in what respect and to what extent function of the heart differs in the patient when compared with a normal person. In both the techniques of electrocardiography and electroencephalography suitable jelly is placed between the electrodes and the skin to ensure good contact. Transistor amplifiers are employed to magnify the very small fifty microvolt waves obtained through the scalp from the surface of the brain when an electroencephalogram record is made. Whenever electrical tracings are taken from the body it is obviously essential to insulate the subject from any other electrical interference.

Four main types of waves are found on an electroencephalogram and tracings from various sites on the scalp are obtained when a record is taken. These are then compared with the typical tracings obtained from a normal person. The wave readings are classified under the letters of the Greek alphabet according to their frequencies.

Alpha waves	8-13	cycles/second
Beta waves	14-30	cycles/second
Delta waves	½-3	cycles/second
Theta waves	4-7	cycles/second

In a normal subject the waves consist of alpha waves when the eyes are closed. When the eyes are opened the alpha rhythm is replaced by small irregular oscillations.

The rhythm recorded in an individual can be modified by a number of factors. For example, when a patient is under an anaesthetic the alpha rhythm is replaced by the beta rhythm. During sleep large waves with a delta rhythm occur. If bright lights are shone on to a subject during an EEG recording or the patient is asked to take several deep breaths then changes in the tracing will occur. Rapid movements of the eyes often occur when a person is asleep and dreaming. The rapid eye movements (R.E.M.) can be picked up by the electrodes and this activity is superimposed on the electroencephalogram tracing.

In monkeys rapid eye movements have been found to occur in the deepest stage of sleep. Investigations on migraine sufferers have revealed that a high proportion of people who wake during the night with a headache have just passed through a period of rapid eye movement on the electroencephalogram. During an epileptic fit changes occur on an electroencephalogram as the seizure is associated with an abnormal discharge of electrical impulses from cells in certain areas of the brain.

An electroencephalogram (EEG) is painless, harmless and relatively inexpensive. It is not, however, a short cut to reaching a diagnosis, as the tracing obtained very rarely points to the definite diagnosis of a condition. In epilepsy, for example, characteristic tracings may be obtained during a fit, but between fits the tracings may be completely normal. In people who suffer from migraine an EEG taken between headache attacks will show differences from the normal in about thirty per cent of migraine sufferers. During a migraine attack this figure rises to about fifty per cent. But here again they are not diagnostic. The cornerstone of diagnosis in both migraine and epilepsy is the account of the disorder which the patient gives to the doctor.

The idea that there might be a link between migraine and epilepsy has been put forward several times over many years. Once the technique of electroencephalography became available it provided a fascinating method of seeing whether or not one could try and link the two conditions. A great deal of work has been done in taking EEG tracings from migraine sufferers. About four per cent of people who suffer from migraine show the same changes that are associated with epilepsy on their EEG. This does not imply that they really suffer from epilepsy or that they ever will. It does suggest, however, that there is some sort of link between the two. Deep breathing exaggerates the changes seen on an EEG tracing.

There is another very interesting link between migraine and epilepsy. Approximately one in three migraine sufferers notice that some of their attacks follow the eating of certain foods. The foods which are mentioned most frequently in relation to migraine attacks are chocolate, cheese and alcohol. As we have already seen cheese contains tyramine which has been shown to precipitate a headache in susceptible subjects. As yet no obvious dietary factors have been implicated in epilepsy but in view of the posible link between migraine and epilepsy studies have been undertaken to see whether or not oral tyramine might produce any changes in the electroencephalogram. These studies were undertaken by research workers at the London Hospital, Whitechapel.

In these studies the help of three groups of volunteers was recruited. One group suffered from migraine but had never noticed any connection between their attacks and anything they had to eat. The second group suffered from migraine but were convinced that when they ate certain foods, notably chocolate, cheese and alcohol, headache attacks became more frequent. The third group suffered from both migraine and epilepsy.

Preliminary EEG records were taken in all the patients in these three groups. These were used as a control or base with which further miligrams records could be compared. Capsules containing one hundred milligrams of tyramine were given to the patients in the three groups and four to seven hours later EEG records were again taken. These records were then looked at by an expert in EEG studies who had no knowledge whatever about the way in which the individual patients had been grouped and what they might have been given to eat. Thus his assessment could only be made on any EEG changes, if such were present, between the original control recordings and those obtained after the tyramine was taken. The findings were of great interest as the records showed significant changes in the EEGs taken after tyramine ingestion in the patients with migraine who linked some of their attacks with food factors and in the patients who suffered from both migraine and epilepsy. More work is being done to investigate these fascinating results further. They imply two things, namely that dietary factors may have some link with epilepsy as well as migraine and they tend to confirm the view that there may also be some sort of link between the biochemical and possibly also vascular changes leading to both conditions.

HEADACHE AND HORMONES

Hormones are chemical messengers which are present in extremely minute amounts in the blood. They have potent and far reaching effects. Everyone for example has heard of the thyroid gland which secretes thyroid hormone. The chief endocrine gland in the body is the pituitary gland, which acts like the leader of an orchestra and influences all the other glands. Despite its major importance in the body it is only the size of a small pea. However, it is very well protected from damage by being situated in a bony hollow in the center of the skull. The pituitary gland produces a number of hormones and influences most of the functions of the body. Some of these hormones, like growth hormone, can act directly on body tissues. Others work by stimulating other endocrine glands, like the ovaries. These other endocrine glands receive the messenger hormones from the pituitary gland and then pour out their own secretion in response. Endocrine glands are ductless glands which release their secretions directly into the blood stream.

The branch of medicine devoted to the study of hormones is called Endocrinology. Our knowledge is rapidly expanding in this area — for example we now know that the cells of the intestinal wall secrete more than 200 differential hormones!

We are thinking about hormones because changes in normal hormonal function can sometimes be associated with headaches. These changes can be considered under a number of different headings.

The menstrual cycle is controlled by a delicate balance of hormones. The average cycle lasts twenty-eight days.

During the first half of each monthly cycle the ovary prepares for the expulsion from its surface of an egg cell or ovum. This passes along the fallopian tube and into the cavity or body of the uterus. This expulsion of the egg or ovum usually occurs around the fourteenth day of the cycle. The lining wall of the uterus then thickens and becomes ready to form a soft bed for the fertilized ovum. This process takes about fourteen days, but if conception has not occurred then this lining is shed after fourteen days with the loss of blood occurring in menstruation. A new cycle then commences.

During the first half of the menstrual cycle the ovary responds to a message sent by the pituitary gland by secreting the hormone estradiol. This is the estrogen which encourages the follicle containing the egg due to be expelled from the ovary to ripen, and midway through the cycle this expulsion of the egg, which is called ovulation, occurs. When ovulation takes place the ovary also starts to secrete another hormone, progesterone. This helps the body of the uterus to prepare itself to receive the egg cell which is about to be expelled. The body of the uterus develops a thickened lining in which the egg cell can embed itself.

If the egg cell is not fertilized then the hormone progesterone gradually ceases to be secreted and after about two weeks it is no longer active. Forty-eight hours after the cessation of progesterone activity the lining membrane of the uterine cavity begins to be shed in the process of menstruation. The hormone estrogen is secreted throughout the whole period of the menstrual cycle, but the level of estrogen also falls at the onset of menstruation.

There is thus a delicate balance between estrogen and

progesterone hormones during the monthly cycle. If conception should occur then the secretion of progesterone continues and menstruation does not occur. The fertilized ovum embeds itself in the thickened wall of the uterus and gradually develops into a fully formed infant.

Progesterone continues to be secreted throughout pregnancy and this is the reason why some women who have previously had repeated miscarriages are treated with injections of progesterone when they become pregnant again. Bleeding can occur when either estrogen or progesterone are suddenly withdrawn. Bleeding due to withdrawal of progesterone and, or estrogen, can occur naturally in the body as in the normal menstrual cycle, or an artificial withdrawal of these hormones can be produced by means of drugs.

If large doses of progesterone are given to a woman during the first half of the menstrual cycle ovulation does not occur. If the administration of progesterone is continued, as in pregnancy, the normal menstrual flow will not occur either. The fact that alterations in the naturally occurring hormonal pattern can inhibit ovulation has led to the introduction of synthetic progesterones for use as oral contraceptives. They are given from the fifth to the twenty-fifth day of the cycle. This use of hormones in women with a normal hormonal cycle is inevitably an interference with the natural pattern of hormone function. In order to reduce the likelihood of bleeding during treatments and to maintain menstrual cycles of normal duration, these synthetic progesterones used as oral contraceptives are supplemented with small amounts of estrogen. Thus oral contraceptives are pills which contain progesterone with varying amounts of estrogen, or pills with progesterone only.

And what bearing does this have on our subject, headache? The increased frequency with which headache occurs in some women in relation to certain phases of the menstrual cycle is well known. These headaches are often migrainous in character.

Some investigators have put the figure for the incidence of migraine in women during their child-bearing years at almost twenty per cent. Migraine attacks which are related to the menstrual cycle occur most commonly either during a menstrual period or in the few days following a period. Progesterone is normally secreted by the ovary from the time of ovulation in the middle of the four week cycle until forty-eight hours before the menstrual flow begins. So migrainous headaches appear to occur mainly at the time when progesterone is not secreted. For this reason treatment with progesterone has been prescribed for women whose headaches occur at this stage of the cycle. Further evidence that progesterone may be an important factor in headaches associated with menstruation is that approximately eighty per cent of migraine sufferers report a spontaneous and complete recovery from migraine during a period of pregnancy. The hormone which is secreted throughout pregnancy is, again, progesterone.

A number of women seem to store water in their bodies at certain times in the monthly cycle, usually just before a period is due to begin. Their waist bands become tighter and their shoes are less comfortable. This water retention is sometimes mentioned by patients as a feature of their migraine attacks. Not infrequently a patient is aware that a migraine attack is about to draw to an end because he or she passes a lot of water. One of the hormones in the body which is concerned with the storage of water is aldosterone. Progesterone seems to have an effect in inhibiting the action both of estrogen and aldosterone and this may be one of the reasons why it helps to alleviate some migraine attacks.

The use of oral contraceptives in the form of the "pill" remains highly controversial. The naturally occurring hormonal cycle demonstrates an extremely delicately balanced mechanism in the body. It is hardly surprising that any interference with this balance results in undesirable side effects. The incidence of headaches in women on the pill is thought to be as high as forty per cent. The other side effects commonly encountered are mood changes, particularly depression, clotting in veins, irregularities in the menstrual cycle and a gain in weight.

An increasing number of young women are being referred to migraine clinics following either an increase in the severity of their headache symptoms or because they have developed migrainous headache as a new symptom since they started on the pill. The pill is given from the fifth to the twenty-fifth day of the menstrual cycle counting the onset of menstruation as the first day of the cycle. Headaches "on the pill" occur most commonly in the intervals between courses.

The headaches which can occur for the first time in women on the pill are often migrainous in nature. This means to say that they are often felt chiefly on one side of the head and are throbbing in character. They may be accompanied by eye signs, nausea and vomiting. The eye signs may consist of blurred vision or flashing lights or zigzag lines, the typical "fortification spectra" may occur. Sometimes the actual head pain is described as "vice-like".

A proportion of the women who complain of headaches when they are taking the pill, possibly about twenty-five per cent of the women who complain of headache, have symptoms which are less characteristic of the typical migraine pattern. Their headaches are felt all over the head and are described as being like a tight band or pressure on the head. They may be accompanied by a feeling of depression or irritability. Sleeplessness may be an associated symptom. These headaches sometimes also occur at the time of the menstrual period.

Very occasionally women who develop headaches on the pill also complain of symptoms associated with a disorder of the nervous system. Among symptoms of this nature that have been reported are loss of sight, usually in one half of the normal field of vision, weakness in an arm or leg or difficulty in speech. These symptoms may last from a few minutes to several hours and are usually temporary although in some rare cases the patient has been left with a permanent defect of vision, or loss of power in a limb. Obviously it is absolutely vital to stop the pill at once in any woman complaining of any symptoms which suggest any disorder of the nervous system. Many physicians and particularly those who work in migraine clinics would go further and consider that the use of the pill is ill advised in any woman who suffers from migraine.

Recent work has shown that the important factor in producing headache in patients taking the pill is the ratio between the amount of estrogen and the amount of progesterone present in the pill. The pill that appears to carry the highest risk in producing unwanted side effects is the one with a high content of estrogen. It has been recommended that only oral contraceptive pills containing less than fifty micrograms of estrogen should be used and this is now standard practice.

Opinions differ, but in my view it is unwise for a migraine sufferer to start taking the pill. Even women who do not suffer from headaches but who have a family history of migraine should embark on this course very warily. If a woman has nevertheless decided to take the pill the danger signals should be heeded carefully. If a patient on the pill starts getting headaches, or if the headaches she already had before she started on the pill become more severe, she should consult her doctor at once. Similarly any symptoms which might be related to damage to the nervous system such as loss of vision, or weakness in a limb should be reported immediately. Even though these symptoms may only last for a few minutes and then recover completely, it is essential to seek medical advice. They should not be ignored under any circumstances.

Every now and then figures are produced for the incidence of headache among women taking the pill. These vary so widely that they are of very little use. The figures differ according to the type of pill being considered and the various criteria for headache adopted by the assessor. The important fact is not the actual figures, which are probably small in relation to the enormous number of women on the pill, but an awareness of its possible harmful effects.

HEADACHE AND HUNGER

We derive our energy from the food that we eat, which provides the fuel that our bodies require to keep running. Starchy food is converted into glucose and this is broken down in the cells of the body to provide energy in the form of heat.

Digestion is the process by which the various foods we eat are broken down by the digestive enzymes or juices into a form which can be absorbed into the bloodstream through the intestinal wall. All carbohydrate or starchy foods such as bread, potatoes, biscuits, cake, sugar and other sweet things are turned into glucose. The digestion of carbohydrates begins in the mouth where a substance in saliva starts breaking down starch. When we eat a starchy meal it takes one to two hours for the carbohydrate to be transformed into glucose and begin to pass into the bloodstream, but if we eat pure glucose the level of glucose in the blood begins to rise within thirty to sixty minutes. In this way pure glucose provides us with a rapid source of energy.

The normal level of glucose in the blood is between eighty and one hundred milligrams per hundred milliliters of blood. If the blood sugar level drops below forty to sixty milligrams per hundred milliliters we feel weak and trembly and tiredness and headaches may occur. In order to investigate the blood sugar level a glucose tolerance curve is obtained. The patient is fasted overnight. In the morning, before any other food is taken, a dose of fifty grams of glucose is given. Small samples of blood are taken from a vein in the arm at half hourly intervals over a two hours period and the glucose content of these blood samples is estimated. A graph is made plotting the glucose content of the blood against the timing of the samples. This is called a glucose tolerance curve.

There are two kinds of glands, those that have ducts and endocrine glands that pour their secretions directly into the blood stream.

The parotid gland is an example of a gland with a duct. This duct opens into the mouth on the inside of the cheek at the level of the upper second molar tooth. The parotid glands become enlarged and painful and the openings of the ducts in the mouth become red and inflamed in mumps.

The pancreas is an example of a gland which has a duct but is also an endocrine gland. The pancreas secretes pancreatic juices which pass through its duct into the small intestine and assist in the breakdown of food in the process of digestion. It also secretes certain hormones directly into the blood stream, the best known of which is insulin.

The way in which the role of the pancreas in glucose metabolism was discovered is interesting. In 1889 two professors in the University of Strasbourg, Von Mering and Minkowski, were studying the part played by the pancreas in the process of digestion. An astute laboratory technician noticed large numbers of flies swarming around the urine of a dog whose pancreas had been removed. He drew attention to this and the urine was found to be loaded with sugar. This chance observation led to the knowledge that the pancreas was concerned in the control of blood sugar levels.

Insulin is essential to glucose metabolism. The glucose level in the blood is regulated by the amount of insulin in the blood. In a healthy person the blood glucose level rises to a level of about one hundred and sixty milligrams in half an hour to an hour after fifty grams of glucose is given orally in a glucose tolerance test. Diabetic subjects suffer from a lack of insulin and because of this much higher blood sugar levels, even exceeding three hundred milligrams per milliliter, may be reached in a glucose tolerance test. The fasting level of blood glucose is also often abnormally high in diabetics. Urine samples are also taken before and during the period of a glucose tolerance test and these are checked for the presence of sugar, not found in the normally healthy person.

The renal threshold level is the blood sugar level at which sugar begins to leak through the kidneys into the urine. The kidneys act as a very delicate filter but sugar does not usually pass from the blood into the urine unless the level in the blood is over one hundred and eighty milligrams per hundred milliliters. Some individuals, however, have a lowered kidney or renal threshold and their kidneys allow sugar to pass from the blood into the urine at a lower blood sugar level. These individuals may have sugar in their urine but a glucose tolerance investigation, which relates the blood sugar level to the sugar present in the urine, shows that their blood sugar levels are within normal limits. Patients with a lowered renal threshold may be losing sugar in the urine but they are not diabetics, since diabetics have raised blood sugar levels. A lowered renal threshold also occurs in some patients during pregnancy.

After it passes into the bloodstream the glucose is dispersed in various ways. Some remains circulating in the body, to provide an immediate source of energy wherever it is required. Some is stored, mainly in the liver, in the form of a substance called glycogen, from which it can readily be converted back into glucose and used for energy if needed. Muscles also store glycogen. Excess glucose, which is not circulating or laid down in glycogen stores, is converted into fat and most of us are well aware of the fat depots in our bodies. When the blood sugar level falls, as in fasting or during heavy exercise, the glycogen is mobilized rapidly and changed back into glucose. In extreme circumstances such as starvation, even fat can be metabolismed into energy.

Every cell in the body requires glucose. Nervous tissue, however, contains no glycogen stores on which to call in an emergency and nervous tissue cells have to rely on glucose carried to them in the blood. If the blood sugar level falls sufficiently low, these nerve cells are deprived of their needs and coma and convulsions may occur. The state in which the blood sugar level falls below the normal fasting blood sugar level of eighty milligrams per hundred milliliters is termed hypoglycemia. This state can occur in such conditions as prolonged fasting, heavy exercise or when a diabetic accidentally has an overdose of insulin.

When the blood sugar level falls some people develop a dull, throbbing headache. Some feel faint and become giddy. This fall in blood sugar occasionally occurs in otherwise fit people who have been eating normally. It sometimes occurs in healthy people between the ages of thirty and forty years, who feel faint, weak and trembly for a short period of time. These symptoms are transient and clear up as soon as a sweet drink is taken.

Some individuals are liable to develop a headache if they miss a regular meal. This is sometimes reported by migraine sufferers. In fact volunteers for migraine research have been asked to fast for a while in order to precipitate an attack. Biochemical studies have then been undertaken both before and during the headache period in an attempt to discover the changes that occur.

There certainly appears to be a link between blood sugar levels and migraine. It has been noted, for example, that when diabetic patients suffer from migraine the attacks of migraine tend to occur when their blood sugar levels are low. The opposite also appears to be true as in the rare instances when a migraine sufferer develops diabetes. It has been noticed that the onset of diabetics with its attendant rise in blood sugar levels has been associated with a diminution in the frequency and severity of migraine attacks. It is also interesting that migraine attacks often become less frequent during pregnancy and during a period of rapid weight gain. In both these states blood sugar levels tend to be on the high side.

Migraine sufferers fairly often report that their attacks begin in the early hours of the morning. It is possible that this timing is associated with the gradual fall in blood sugar level overnight following an evening meal. It is simple enough for any migraine sufferer whose attacks frequently commence in the early hours of the morning to test this hypothesis by taking a sugary drink last thing at night. By the time the sufferer wakes with a headache, however it may be too late to prevent the chain of events. Precautionary measures are worth trying so keep a glucose drink by the bedside.

In a similar way we can try to apply our knowledge about blood sugar levels in migraine to help other headache sufferers. There are, of course, the obvious measures. Individuals who tend to develop a headache if they miss a meal should be extra careful about eating at regular intervals. If a journey has to be undertaken, or a shopping expedition, or anything that might interfere with a mealtime, arrangements should be made to carry a sugary drink or to take glucose sweets.

Young people sometimes develop headaches during or after active exercise such as running or playing football. We know that muscles use up some of their stores of glycogen during exercise. A drink, sweetened with glucose, before and during a period of exertion may prove helpful.

The reproductive hormones and insulin are the hormones which most often have a bearing on the incidence of headache. Headaches sometimes occur in patients with a high blood pressure, which can be secondary to hormonal changes. Other hormonal causes of headache are rare.

HEADACHE AND ALLERGY

I do not like you, Doctor Fell,
The reason why I cannot tell,
But this alone, I know full well,
I do not like you, Doctor Fell.

John Fell was Dean of Christ Church in Oxford in the middle of the seventeenth century. He pardoned a student about to be expelled from the University when the student gave an unprepared translation of a Latin epigram in the words quoted above. Poor Dr. Fell was disliked by the students for no apparent reason. It may, of course, have had something to do with the fact that he restored law and order to the University after a period in which anarchy had reigned!

In allergic states the body takes a dislike, and reacts, for no obvious reason to a substance to which it has become sensitive. Allergy is a word with which we are all familiar. We hear it almost every day in general conversation and it is universally recognised as a state in which contact with a substance causes unpleasant physical effects.

The term allergy is often used loosely but medically speaking it is a state in which the body reacts to a foreign protein, called an antigen or allergen by producing antibodies. A number of different types of antibody have been identified and their levels in the blood can be estimated by techniques used in the science of immunology.

Transplant surgery has resulted in an enormous concentration of interest in immunology. When an organ, such as a kidney, is transplanted it can act as a foreign protein or allergen and the body of the recipient reacts to it and may even reject it. In order for a transplant to be successful the tissues of the donor and the recipient have to match extremely closely.

Blood contains both red cells and white cells, and it is a certain type of white cell that is responsible for the production of antibodies. The antibodies are made of immunoglobulins which are derived from the gamma globulin fraction of proteins. Antibodies or immunoglobulins are identified both by their structure and their function. Thus the largest immunoglobulin is termed IgM, or Ig macroglobulin. This comprises 8% of the immuno globulin normally present in the body. Owing to its large molecular size it remains in the blood stream, where it provides the first line of defense against bacterial infections. Patients who have a deficiency of IgM may suffer from recurrent bacterial infections. IgA is found in the gut wall and other body spaces and a deficiency of IgA leads to increased respiratory and digestive tract disorders. A number of immunoglobulins have been identified but the one in which we are particularly interested is IgE.

IgE is concerned in the typical allergic reaction and the levels of IgE in the blood rise with an allergic reaction.

An allergic reaction produces swelling, inflammation and destruction of tissue. We have all come across people who develop a highly irritating rash, looking rather like a large number of inflamed blisters, whenever they eat shell fish or strawberries. This is called urticaria. An allergic reaction may be localised to a small area of the body or it may be generalized. A bee sting provides an example of a localized allergic reaction. The bee injects a foreign protein into the skin and the surrounding area reacts by becoming red, hot and swollen. Serum sickness is an example of a generalized reaction. Serum is occasionally given to patients when they are innoculated against certain diseases. On rare occasions the body reacts to this serum. About a week after the serum is given a slight rise in temperature occurs and swelling of the joints and a rash develop. Usually this all settles down within a few days.

Probably the allergen with which we are all most familiar is pollen. An allergic reaction to pollen is so common that some newspapers give a daily pollen count during the hay fever season. A count consists of the number of pollen grains from grasses per cubic meter of air, averaged over twenty-four hours. At fifty or more, hay fever sufferers are likely to have severe symptoms. A large number of people suffer from asthma and hay fever and in both of these disorders many sufferers are aware of the substances which may trigger off their attacks. These are frequently inhalants such as pollen or house dust but certain foods have also been implicated.

Skin tests are sometimes used in order to see whether or not a sufferer from hay fever or asthma is sensitive to a particular substance. They have only very rarely been found to be of any help in assessing the causes of migraine. Skin tests are carried out in the following way. The skin of the smooth surface of the forearm is the site usually chosen for these tests. The area is cleaned very carefully with a substance that will not cause any skin reaction. Small breaks are then made in the skin surface without drawing any blood. One such area is left to act as a control with which the other areas can be compared. Into the other broken areas various agents are gently rubbed. These agents are substances like pollen or horse dander which are suspected of being concerned in producing some of the attacks of asthma or hay fever or whatever condition we are investigating. A chart is carefully made identifying the various skin areas and labelling them with the agents used. The whole site is then observed to see whether any changes occur which make any of the broken areas on which suspected agents have been applied look any different from the control area. If the person being tested is sensitive to any agent the appropriate area is likely to show a change within an hour or so. The area becomes slightly swollen and inflamed. The patient is asked to observe the skin site for a period of up to twenty-four hours and to report if any further changes occur. If any particular substance produces a reaction its role in the disorder being treated can then be investigated.

Allergy to cow's milk, for example, has been found to be responsible for 25% of the cases of asthma in childhood. Childhood eczema, colic and rhinitis are sometimes also attributed to this allergy. Food additives such as tartrazine, a yellow colouring agent, and sodium benzoate, an antibacterial and antifungal agent, can also cause asthma. Mouth ulcers can result from an allergy to gluten, tomatoes and potatoes.

In recent years a great deal of interest has been focussed on the possible role of foods in mental illness, particularly cereals and the gluten contained in wheat, barley and lentils. Dramatic improvement has been reported in mentally ill patients treated with a cereal free diet. If these reports are confirmed they will obviously be of tremendous importance.

In the past the term allergy was used to cover a wide variety of medical conditions whose causes were poorly understood. Migraine has often been included among the allergic disorders and in the first half of this century a great deal was written about this aspect of the disorder. Migraine resembles allergic states like asthma and hay fever because like them, it arises at intervals and in a paroxysmal way. The fact that a proportion of migraine sufferers link the incidence of their attacks with the eating of certain foods was one of the chief reasons why migraine was considered an allergic condition.

It is difficult without introducing an allergic factor, to understand why some migraine sufferers associate some of their attacks with the inhalation of certain substances. .The inhalants most commonly mentioned are tobacco smoke, paint, perfume and house dusts. During an allergic reaction various substances are released in the body, which might affect the size of blood vessels. They are called vasoactive amines and they could be a factor in the production of headache, but a great deal of research needs to be done in this area before any positive statements could be made.

Interest in headache and allergy has been concentrated largely in the area of headache precipitating foods. Scientifically speaking, however, we have to restrict the term allergy to conditions in which there is a detectable immunological reaction in the body. Recent research has shown that the foods implicated in headache often contain pharmacologically active substances which act directly on a tissue of the body without involving antibodies or any other allergic response. For example alcoholic drinks and certain cheeses contain pharmacologically active substances which have an effect on the size of blood vessels. It is their ability to do this which causes their headache producing effects.

Again, some people appear to be extra sensitive to the caffeine content of coffee, particularly when it is taken in excess. A state of anxiety, palpitations, headache and gastro-intestinal symptoms may occur. The "Chinese restaurant" syndrome comes into the same category. Here there is a sensitivity to monosodium glutamate which is used as a preservative, and the patient may fail to finish his meal because of a feeling of tightness in his chest and across his upper arms and face and headache.

The way in which the eating of certain foods can be linked with headache is dealt with more fully in the chapter on Headache and Food.

HEADACHES AND FOOD

"Milk is not recommended for those who
suffer from headaches.
Cheese . . . is not equally harmful to all
Sweet wine is less likely to produce
headache than is heavy wine."
                              Hippocratic Writings

Over two thousand years ago Hippocrates drew attention to the link between certain foods and headache. In the eighteenth century an eminent British physician, John Fothergill, wrote a classic treatise on the same subject. Fothergill, who was a Quaker, was born in 1712. He was not only a great physician but a good man, active in prison reform, the abolition of slavery and the improvement of medical education. It is of interest that he refused to accept an appointment as a Royal physician. Fothergill is said to have worked 16 or 17 hours a day, often going for 24 hours without sleep. As a Quaker he had many friends in America, particularly in Philadelphia and he gave a large sum of money to the Pennsylvania Hospital before he died at the age of 68 years.

Fothergill wrote:

"There are some things which, in very small quantities, seldom fail to produce the sick headache in some constitutions. Such are a larger proportion than usual of melted butter, fat meats, and spices, especially common black pepper. Meat pies often contain all these things united, and are as fertile a cause of this complaint as any thing I know; so are rich baked puddings, and every thing of a similar nature. A little error in these things will seldom fail to be attended with much suffering, in many constitutions."

During the next two hundred years a number of well documented observations have been made on the relationship between the head and the stomach. When the subject of headaches and food is discussed we would do well to heed the wise words of Edward Liveing. He spent a lifetime studying the subject of headache and published an authoritative work "On Megrim, Sick-Headache and Some Allied Disorders" in 1873. He commented

"One way in which traditional error in such matters is propagated is, I am convinced, in many cases, by our faulty methods of interrogation. On the one hand, we are too apt to accept in the hurry of routine the inferences of patients for statements of fact; and on the other, we often wring from them conformity to our views by pressing them with leading questions or anticipating what they have to say.

This is an area in which I have been particularly interested myself and I asked 500 migraine sufferers who thought that some of their attacks were sometimes linked with the eating of certain foods, which foods they avoided eating for this reason. The food which these 500 dietary migraine sufferers cited in order of frequency were:

Chocolate	75%
Cheese and diary products	48%
Citrus fruits	30%
Alcoholic drinks	25%
Fatty fried food	18%
Vegetables especially onions	18%

Tea and coffee	14%
Meat especially pork	14%
Sea food	10%

Although approximately one third of all migraine sufferers relate the incidence of some of their attacks to the eating of certain foods this does not mean that food is the only factor responsible for headaches in these patients. All the other possible causes of migraine may also be operating but in addition these sufferers have learned through experience to beware of eating certain foods.

There are of course other migraine sufferers, who are unaware that the eating of some foods may be related to some of their attacks. If doubt exists, it is worth noting what a migraine sufferer has eaten in the twenty-four hours before an attack. To become a food faddist may be as great a burden to a migraine sufferer, not to mention his friends and family, as suffering from occasional headaches. But without going to any extremes every migraine sufferer should be aware of the foods which might possibly be involved. It is simple to have a trial period of say six weeks, and exclude chocolate, cheese and alcohol, which are the most common precipitants, from the diet. The effect of excluding citrus fruits and coffee may also occasionally be rewarding. A trial period may prove particularly helpful in the treatment of severe and frequent attacks where the sufferer may be totally unaware of the fact that daily drinks containing chocolate or cheese sandwiches are maintaining a cycle of headaches.

Migraine is a disorder in which changes occur during an attack in the size of blood vessels in the head. The foods that sometimes precipitate migraine contain certain substances, called amines, which are capable of affecting blood vessel size. The way in which these vasoactive amines act in producing headaches is described in the section of this book on headache and chemistry. The vasoactive amines which are found in headache precipitating foods include β-phenylethylamine, octopamine and histamine, as well as tyramine.

Tyramine is found particularly in substances which have undergone bacterial decomposition such as game and certain cheeses. The amount of tyramine present is not constant to any particular cheese. The tyramine content of cheese ranges from approximately one hundred milligrams in four ounces of a cheddar cheese rich in tyramine to trace amounts or none in other cheeses. Even in one specific type of cheese the amount of tyramine present varies according to the maturation time of the cheese, the bacterial flora and details of manufacture. It is not related to the flavour or appearance of the cheese. The cheeses in which the highest content of tyramine have been found are Stilton, Cheddar and blue cheese. As the tyramine content of even the same brand of cheese varies greatly a susceptible person might eat a particular sort of cheese with impunity on several successive occasions before having any reaction to its tyramine content.

Tyramine, however, is by no means the only constituent of foods which can precipitate a headache. Chocolate contains dozens of amines, some of which have vasoactive properties similar to those of tyramine. One which is present in very small amounts in chocolate, but found in large amounts in cheese and certain alcoholic drinks, is β-phenylethylamine. This substance has been tested in a pure form in a controlled trial in selected migraine sufferers and has been shown to act as a headache precipitant.

Octopamine is a vasoactive amine present in citrus fruits. Clinical observations suggest that when large amounts of pure orange or lemon juice are taken headache may occasionally result. This is probably due to the action of octopamine.

Certain cheeses and other foodstuffs which have a high content of protein-splitting bacteria also have a high content of histamine. The formation of histamine in the intestinal tract depends on the presence of histidine in the diet. The histidine content of food is roughly proportional to its protein content, as histidine is an amino-acid found in many proteins. White wines may contain up to ten milligrams of histamine per liter and in some red wines this figure rises to twenty milligrams per liter.

There is one type of headache which is known to be related to histamine, cluster headache. The pain of cluster headache is usually felt around one eye and may last from a few minutes to a few hours. The eye on the affected side of the head becomes reddened, puffy and watery and the nostril on that side often feels blocked. The interesting point is that during a susceptible phase, when a patient is suffering from recurring attacks of pain, a number of substances are capable of triggering off the painful symptoms. Chief among these substances is histamine. Among others are alcohol and nitroglycerine. It would seem that during a time when cluster headaches are recurring the blood vessels of these sufferers are susceptible to the action of substances which affect blood vessels, and that at such times these substances trigger headache attacks.

The role of histamine in cluster headache is undisputed. If a person, even a person who does not usually get headaches, is given an intravenous injection of one tenth of a milligram of histamine acid phosphate, a generalized throbbing headache will result. If histamine is given in the same way to a migraine sufferer during an attack then the pain on the side of the head which is already painful becomes much worse. Instead of producing the generalized headache that occurs in normal people, histamine exaggerates the headache on the already painful area of the head on a migraine attack.

Two types of metabolism occur in the body. These are termed exogenous and endogenous. Exogenous metabolism occurs when a substance is taken into the body, such as glucose by mouth. Endogenous metabolism of glucose would occur when glycogen is broken down in the liver to form glucose. Both types of metabolism occur constantly in relation to various substances. The end products of both endogenous and exogenous metabolism may result in the excretion of substances in the urine. Histamine excretion has been found to be increased in some patients with migraine and in some patients with cluster headache. This is probably due to an altered form of endogenous metabolism. The main breakdown product of histamine in the urine is 1.4-methyl imidazole acetic acid. The amount of this substance in the urine has also been found to be increased in some migraine sufferers even between attacks.

Gastrointestinal Factors

A number of headache sufferers feel convinced that their headaches are closely linked with their digestion. Some migraine patients have also reported an alteration in the frequency of their attacks during a period when they have been taking antibiotic medicines. These observations lead one to consider whether there are factors operating in the alimentary tract that have an influence on the incidence of headaches.

It is highly likely that this is the case. The use of antibiotics affects the bacterial flora in the intestine. Whether we like it or not our intestines are teaming with living organisms which are largely concerned with the breakdown of food products passing through. When this passage of food is slowed, as in constipation, or altered by changes in the bacterial flora concerned in its breakdown, increased putrefaction or decarboxylation may occur. Once again we are back with our now familiar amines. They are formed in increased amounts when the process of digestion is slowed and vasoactive amines such as tyramine may be produced in increased amounts and be absorbed in the bloodstream. Toxic effects like headache may result from this.

Food substances like yoghurt have a high content of bacterial flora. If you eat a lot of yoghurt this could affect your intestinal content of organisms and the process of food breakdown. An excessively rapid passage of food through the intestine may also precipitate headache. This can occur with the excessive use of laxatives.

Food Additives

Sodium Nitrite. There have been reports of patients

who developed headaches after eating frankfurter sausages. The active constituent in the sausages which are found to be responsible for the headaches was sodium nitrite. This substance is also present in cured meat products such as bacon, salami and ham. Ten milligrams of sodium nitrite has been shown to provoke headaches in susceptible individuals.

Sodium Glutamate is used as a preservative in a number of foods. It was the agent responsible for symptoms occurring in the "Chinese restaurant Syndrome". These symptoms occurred 15 to 25 minutes after a meal and consisted of a burning sensation in the back of the neck, across the front of the chest and over the forearms, together with a tightness across the chest. As little as 5 gm. of sodium glutamate could produce this effect.

Tartrazine. This is an orangy yellow powder which makes a golden yellow solution. It is a useful coloring agent for medicines and is used as a dye in some foods. As little as 1 to 2 mg. can sometimes give rise to asthma, urticaria and occasionally headache in susceptible individuals.

Caffeine

The fact that coffee drinking can keep some of us awake at night is well known. Coffee can also have other ill-effects and medical reports have drawn attention to the fact that caffeine, which is the chief active ingredient of coffee beans, could well be one of the more frequent causes of chronic recurrent headaches. Excessive coffee drinking can also give rise to a number of other symptoms such as irritability, tremulousness, occasional muscle twitching and palpitations.

Caffeine is present not only in coffee but also in other common drinks such as tea and coca cola. The surprising thing is that while ground coffee beans contain about 1 to 2% of caffeine, tea can contain as much as 4%, and there may be about 60 mg of caffeine in a small cup of strong tea. Instant coffee has a caffeine content of approximately 3 to 4%.

When caffeine is used medicinally it is given in doses of 100 mg to 300 mg. It is easy to see how rapidly one can exceed the maximum dose if one drinks more than a pint of coffee or tea!

Caffeine is a stimulant and is contained in a number of analgesic tablets used particularly in the treatment of headache. It is also present in some preparations for migraine where it is thought to enhance the action of ergotamine. It is only sensible to look at the formula on the box of any analgesic tablets that you are taking for headache symptoms. Three tablets containing 30 mg of caffeine may well keep you awake at night, if taken late in the day.

Ice Cream Headache

Headache sometimes occurs when very cold foods touch the palate. This is thought to happen more often in migraine sufferers than in other people and is possibly due to the effect of extreme cold on nervous reflexes. Not surprisingly the food most often associated with this type of headache is ice cream.

Alcohol

As far as headaches are concerned alcoholic drinks contain several substances that must be regarded with suspicion. To start with they contain ethyl alcohol. This causes blood vessels on the surface of the body to dilate. The rosy flush which follows one or two glasses of wine as well as the red face of the chronic alcoholic are visible evidence of this. We have already seen that in people who suffer from migraine the blood vessels which are affected in an attack appear to react in a particularly sensitive way to any stimuli. The action of alcohol in dilating blood vessels could be such a stimulus. It is not only migraine sufferers who get a headache after alcohol. The difference is really one of degree. The typical hangover headache is due to vasodilation and usually occurs after a considerable amount of alcohol has been taken. Some migraine sufferers develop an attack after drinking relatively small amounts of alcohol.

When large amounts of alcohol are taken a fall in the level of blood sugar occurs. This, too, could act as a precipitating factor in headache.

Alcoholic drinks often contain several of the vasoactive amines that have already been mentioned in connection with headache. Chief of these are tyramine, histamine and betaphenylethylamine.

The common use of the breathalyzer in our everyday life focusses interest on the facts and figures related to alcohol consumption. The breathalyzer is a portable instrument which measures the amount of alcohol in exhaled air. The breathalyzer test alone cannot be used as evidence in court and blood and urine samples are also taken if the crystals in the breathalyzer change colour, thus indicating that the content of alcohol in the exhaled air is high. In Britain it is an offense for a driver to be in charge of a vehicle when his blood alcohol level exceeds 80 mg. per 100 ml. or if the urine level exceeds 107 mg. per 100 ml. Stupor occurs with a blood alcohol level of 300 mg. per 100 ml. of blood. A significant increase in the accident rate has been found with levels of 40 to 50 mg. per 100 ml. and when the level reaches 100 mg. per 100 ml. the probability of causing an accident rises 6 to 7 fold that of a driver with a level less than 10 mg per 100 ml. With a blood level of 150 mg. per 100 ml. the probability of an accident is increased 25 fold.

Thus those who abstain from alcohol because it gives them a headache, often long before the breathalyzer danger level, may be forunate in having an effective built-in warning system!

HEADACHE IN CHILDREN

The incidence of headache in children is surprisingly high. One would, of course, expect headache symptoms to occur in association with the onset of the common infections of childhood, such as measles and chicken pox. One would also understand headaches arising in children with rare conditions such as meningitis. But one might well be amazed to learn that a number of surveys have revealed that by the early age of seven years, roughly one in three children gives a history of headaches.

Like the most common type of headache in adults, the most common type of headache to occur in childhood is tension headache. Tension, of course, can arise at any age and results in the contraction of muscles in the head and neck which produces pain. While children suffer from tension in the same way as adults, children are often inarticulate and unable to express their anxieties and fears. They can become very worried over matters to which no adult would give a second thought and considerable perception may be needed to discern them. For example, a child may find reading difficult and become so anxious on a day when he thinks that he might be asked to read aloud at school that a headache develops.

Tension headache in children is frequently described as a painful tightness all around the head. Nausea and vomiting are rare in tension headache. The treatment lies in determining the cause and trying to deal with it as far as possible. Patience, love and understanding will go a lot further in treating this type of headache than criticism, pills and potions.

Two types of headache commonly encountered in children have been mentioned. These are the headaches which accompany acute infections and tension headache. The third type of headache which occurs fairly commonly in childhood is vascular which means that the pain is accompanied by changes in the size of blood vessels. Children do not suffer from disorders of blood vessels such as temporal arteritis. Cluster headache, has, however, been reported on rare occasion at an early age. Migraine is a vascular headache.

Migraine is very rare in early childhood. At five years the incidence is only one per cent or less. By the age of eleven it has risen to about five per cent in both sexes although the figure varies according to where the survey is taken. At all events the incidence of migraine in girls rises sharply during the teenage years.

Migraine is classified into two types, common and classical. In both, headache, nausea and frequently vomiting occur. In classical migraine the symptoms of common migraine are preceded by warning signs. These most often affect eyesight and are called an aura. Common migraine is found more often than classical migraine in both boys and girls. Classical migraine is found more often in girls than boys.

Periodic bouts of vomiting, travel and car sickness are common in children and are sometimes forerunners of the migraine attacks which start a few years later. This is particularly the case in families where one or other parent has migraine or where there is a strong family history of migraine since migraine is a familial disorder. Migraine in the young is often associated with severe nausea and vomiting and the headache usually affects both sides of the head. The attacks are periodic and may be preceded by some of the warning symptoms that herald an attack of classical migraine, such as visual disturbances. Sometimes these attacks are associated with periods of confusion which pass off as the symptoms improve. Dizziness and a staggering gait occasionally accompany the headache symptoms.

Any doctor who is examining a young child with headache symptoms will take a very careful history from the parents and will want to do two things without fail. He will measure the size of the child's head to see whether this is appropriate for the child's expected development at that age. he will use an ophthalmoscope to look into the back of the eye and see whether there are any signs of pressure inside the skull. This can be seen by inspecting the flat white disc at the back of the eye. This disc is the flattened head of the optic nerve, the edges of which become blurred with increased pressure. Less frequently an X-ray of the skull or the much rarer brain scan investigation may prove helpful in addition to a routine examination. An electroencephalogram (EEG) is also sometimes helpful when the possibility of epilepsy is being considered in children with recurrent fits or faints.

Before passing on to the treatment of headache in children one has to remember that children are commonly falling and bumping their heads. This can produce neuralgic pain which may be felt in the back of the head.

Abdominal Migraine

This is a rare variant of migraine in which the attacks of pain in the head are replaced by recurrent attacks of abdominal pain. This pain may be associated with nausea and vomiting and it is only its recurrence in the absence of any abnormal physical findings, in a patient with a family history of migraine, that eventually leads the physician to the correct diagnosis. Like migraine in childhood it is a diagnosis which can only be arrived by a process of exclusion. Abdominal migraine is interesting in so far as the symptoms appear to respond more readily to anticonvulsant therapy, than to other drugs usually used in the treatment of migraine.

The term "periodic syndrome" has been used to describe a particular group of recurrent symptoms which are recognized in school-children. This term covers a number of symptoms which can be divided up in the following way in order to give you a rough idea about their relative frequency in children of school age:

1 in 10	Abdominal pain
1 in 7	Headache
1 in 25	Limb pain

This "periodic syndrome" includes the disorder referred to as "cyclical vomiting" in which vomiting and abdominal pain recur at intervals. Children who suffer from the "periodic syndrome" sometimes develop migraine later on in life. Occasionally recurrent pains in the arms or legs, in fact typical "growing pains" are the only signs of the periodic syndrome in children.

Treatment

The most important thing to do for children with headache is to ensure that a correct diagnosis is made, for example, if a mother suffers from migraine herself and her child starts having headaches she should let a doctor see the child and decide upon the treatment. It would be quite wrong if the parents assumed the child had a migraine, like its mother and failed to get treatment for some other causes of the pain, such as ear or tooth trouble, which is then neglected.

Obvious measures such as ensuring that the child has adequate sleep and regular meals may be obvious but are often overlooked. Common sense should be the first priority in the treatment of children with headaches. In the treatment of tension headache in children the most important factor is the understanding and cooperation of the child's parents.

Possible precipitating causes of migraine should be

recognized and excluded. These include stress, irregular meals and occasionally dietary factors such as chocolate, cheese and citrus fruits.

Very often a mild sedative such as small doses of valium for a few weeks is all that is needed to reduce the frequency and severity of the headaches. Where further treatment is necessary ordinary analgesics such as soluble aspirin are the best way to tackle the problem. When a headache begins it is vital to give the analgesic as soon as possible. Trouble sometimes arises with children at school who develop a headache during school hours. They may be too shy to explain to the teacher that they are getting a headache and several hours can pass before they get home. By then it is too late for any tablets to be effective. For this reason it is a good idea for the mother of a child with migraine to speak to the teacher and explain the position. The child can then take a suitable tablet to school and be encouraged to take it as soon as a headache begins.

If relatively simple measures taken to control migraine attacks in children are ineffective then other drugs may be prescribed by the physician. These include drugs such as Cyproheptadine hydrochloride 4 mg. a day at bedtime and more rarely Propanolol 10 to 20 mg daily as preventive therapy in migraine. Chlordiazepoxide (Librium) in doses of 10 mg. twice daily has few side effects and can be helpful. Where thc EEG investigation has revealed any abnormality of rhythm drugs such as Phenytoin (Epanutin) may prove helpful in preventing migraine attacks.

HEADACHE AND BLOOD PRESSURE

As we grow older our blood pressure tends to rise slightly. Most of us have had our blood pressure taken at one time or another. An inflatable cuff is wrapped around the upper part of an arm and air is pumped into it. At the same time the pressure inside the inflatable cuff is recorded by means of a column of mercury. The doctor places his stethoscope on an artery which runs down the upper arm and in front of the elbow, and listens to the dull thud in this brachial artery which is heard every time the heart beats and pushes blood along it. When the artery is so compressed by the inflatable cuff that the pressure of the cuff obstructs blood flowing along the artery, the sound made by the heart beat is no longer heard. The pressure in the cuff at this cut off point is recorded by noting how high the column of mercury has risen. This reading is normally 100 mm of mercury plus the age of the person — so in a man or woman of 40 years it would normally be 140 mm of mercury. The air is then slowly allowed to escape from the inflatable cuff. Not only does the person whose blood pressure is being recorded sense the welcome return of blood flow to his arm and hand but the doctor hears the beats again as blood is propelled through the artery with each heart beat. But even when the heart is not actually contracting there is blood in the artery. This blood maintains a constant pressure in the artery and when this constant pressure level is reached the beats cease to be heard through the stethoscope. This constant pressure should be around 80 to 90 mm of mercury and this reading forms the second or lower blood pressure reading. So we can take it that the normal blood pressure is around 100 + age over 80 to 90 mm of mercury. The upper recording is called the systolic pressure while the lower is the diastolic. Patients with a raised blood pressure sometimes complain of a headache. Typically this is felt in the early morning when the patient wakes up, and it is usually most marked across the back of the head.

It is often relieved if the patient takes things quietly and sits up in bed gradually and has a cup of tea before getting up. When the diastolic blood pressure rises above 140 mm of mercury then chronic headache occurs, but with the excellent therapy now available for the treatment of a high blood pressure this state of affairs should only very rarely arise, and when it does there is a need for immediate treatment.

If you are being treated for a raised blood pressure or consult your doctor because you are suffering from headaches, then he is likely to examine your eyes with an ophthalmoscope. This instrument enables the doctor to look through the pupil of the eye and study the blood vessels running across the retina at the back of the eye. These blood vessels are terminal branches of the internal carotid artery. They show characteristic changes if the blood pressure rises and remains raised. They are therefore very helpful in indicating what is going on in the blood vessels in other parts of the body since the back of the eye is the only place where one can actually obtain a direct view of blood vessels.

If headache symptoms are due to a raised blood pressure then they should improve as the blood pressure falls to normal levels with treatment.

HEADACHE AND THE KIDNEY

Transplant surgery has provided some of the most dramatic advances in modern medicine. While the subject of heart transplants remains an open issue kidney transplants have become an acceptable method for the treatment of certain kidney diseases. The fact that kidney transplants are not undertaken more frequently than they are at present is due not to a lack of patients but to a lack of donor kidneys. Why are our kidneys so vital to life and what function do they perform?

A living cell is in a constant state of activity. In order to maintain this activity, in fact in order to maintain life, a ceaseless turnover of essential materials occurs in the cells. These materials are carried to them in the bloodstream. Waste products are inevitably formed in the cells and these need to be eliminated from the body. They are carried by the blood to the kidneys, which act primarily as a filtering system.

The functional unit of the kidney is the nephron, of which each human kidney contains about one million. Each nephron is formed from two parts. There is a coiled globular shaped part called a glomerulus and a long tubule

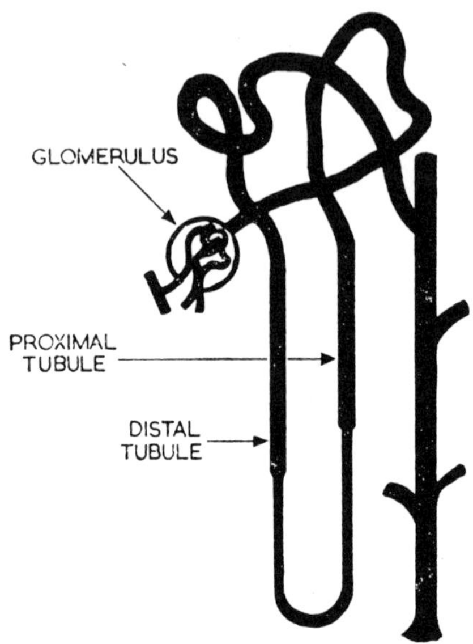

Diagram of nephron.

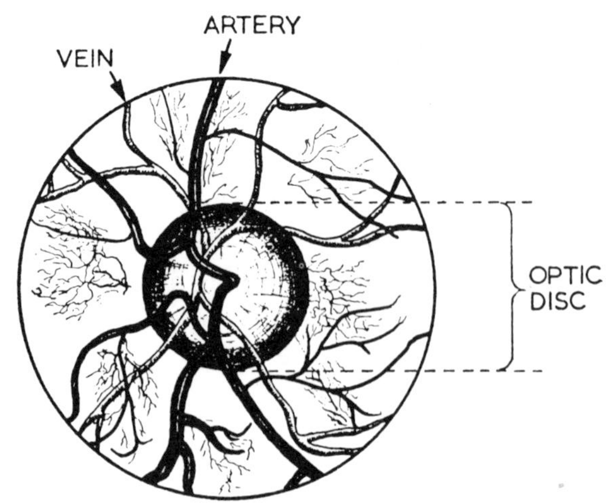

The view through an ophthalmoscope.

which is arranged in loop formation. Blood consists of a liquid portion or plasma, in which are suspended the different cells, red cells, white cells and platelets. Dissolved in the blood are various salts, organic substances, hormones, vitamins, the products of repair and breakdown in the body, antibodies and enzymes. The function of the kidney is to regulate normal concentrations of the constituents of the blood, by the excretion of water, the soluble end products of nitrogen metabolism and the electrolytes necessary to maintain the electrolyte balance of the blood.

The glomeruli of the kidney work extremely hard. Each glomerulus consists of a tuft of minute capillary channels supplied individually by the terminal branches of the renal artery which brings blood to the kidney. The glomerulus is enclosed in a capsule. In a period of twenty-four hours the glomeruli filter approximately 170 to 200 liters of protein free fluid from the blood. This means that they filter about fifty to sixty times the volume of plasma in the blood.

As the amount of urine that we pass on average during the day is one and a half liters it is obvious that extensive reabsorption of the fluid filtered by the glomeruli occurs. This reabsorption takes place in the tubules. They return to the bloodstream those substances which the body needs while waste products are left to pass out into the urine. The end-product of protein metabolism in the body is urea. This is formed in the liver and about two thirds of the urea produced in the body is excreted through the kidneys. The concentration of urea in the blood is normally between twenty to forty milligrams per hundred milliliters. The average daily excretion of urea is from twenty-five to thirty-five grams.

Not only do the kidneys deal with the waste products of metabolism in the body but they maintain the pH or hydrogen ion concentration of the blood at a constant level. The blood is very slightly alkaline with a pH of 7.4.

If the kidney fails to function efficiently certain substances accumulate in the blood, chiefly urea. Urea is the end-product of the breakdown of protein which goes on constantly in the living cell. Very often a failure of kidney function is temporary and can be treated by extremely careful dietary measures which consist chiefly in the restriction of protein intake. If the kidney failure persists, however, the body gradually becomes poisoned by the accumulation of its own breakdown products.

There are two ways of dealing with this failure of kidney function when it poses a long-term problem. Renal transplant surgery provides one method of replacing a kidney which can no longer function adequately by a healthy kidney from a suitable donor. The emphasis is on the word suitable, as very careful matching of the recipient and donor tissues is essential. The method more commonly used to treat a failure of kidney function is renal dialysis. The body of the patient is connected to a machine which acts like an artificial kidney and filters the waste products out of the blood by passing it through various semipermeable layers. This restores the blood of the patient to a normal healthy state. The process of renal dialysis using an artificial kidney machine usually takes several hours. It is frequently carried out overnight. In this way sufferers from severe kidney disease can be kept well and at work. The chief problem, at present, is the lack of adequate numbers of kidney machines.

The reason why the subject of renal dialysis is included in a book on headache is that about two thirds of the patients who undergo treatment with an artificial kidney machine develop a headache during the procedure. This may be migrainous in character and usually occurs one to nine hours after the start of treatment. The peak incidence is between four and seven hours.

The symptom of headache has been reported only in patients who still retain their diseased kidney or kidneys. If the diseased kidneys are removed and their function taken over by an artificial kidney machine then the headaches do not seem to occur. Kidney disease is sometimes associated with a raised blood pressure. Possibly the patient's blood pressure rises a little just before a treatment on the artificial kidney machine is due as the headache appears to be linked with the fall in blood pressure which may accompany treatment.

Treatment with an artificial kidney machine has given a new lease of life to many sufferers from kidney disease, and headache may seem a relatively small price to pay for the benefits obtained. Nevertheless anyone who has ever had a severe headache will feel acute sympathy with the sufferers on renal dialysis. However, because the changes in their blood are very closely monitored during treatment with an artificial kidney machine it may prove possible to pinpoint the factors associated with the occurrence of headache. This knowledge could eventually lead to adequate preventive measures during renal dialysis. It could also prove of eventual benefit to other headache sufferers.

HEADACHE AND TEETH

It was Mark Twain who commented that Adam and Eve had many advantages but the principal one was that they escaped teething! Our teeth are a source of trouble to many of us not only in the cradle but to the grave, if they last that long. There can be very few who do not know what toothache feels like. And it is not only our teeth that can cause trouble. Occasionally the jaw, too, can give rise to pain. This has sometimes been confused with migraine and other types of headache and must be carefully differentiated from them.

We have all been told at one time or another to grit our teeth and get on with it! This advice implies several things. First of all it suggests that we are facing an unwelcome situation. We are anxious about it and need to make a determined effort to overcome it. It also implies that when we are anxious we often make a physical as well as a mental effort to cope with a problem. We associate tension in our muscles with mental tension. If you are sitting in a chair waiting for an important interview you are unlikely to lean back in an easy relaxed manner. You are more likely to be perched alert and upright at the edge of the chair with every muscle taut. In some patients, especially those who are depressed or worried, this tension may affect the muscles of the jaw so much that it occasionally results in pain. This pain may be associated with toothgrinding, and tension in the muscles of the back of the head and neck can result in tension headache. Pain may be felt in the back of the neck, the temples and the top of the head as well as in the jaw joint.

Anxiety and tension, however, are not essential features of pain in the jaw. Some patients have a faulty bite. When they close their jaws the upper and lower jaw joint are out of alignment when the teeth are clenched. Clicking of the jaw may be an indication of this. The upper teeth may also slide on the lower teeth when the jaw is closed. Occasionally faulty alignment of the jaw joint occurs after one or more of the molar teeth at the back of the mouth are extracted. The upper and lower jaws are affected by the gap and no longer meet smoothly. This trouble can also arise in a patient with dentures. It is given the name Bruxism or Myofacial pain dystropy (MPD).

Patients with trouble of this nature usually complain of pain on one side of the head in or near the ear. The muscle over the jaw joint may be painful to pressure. Clicking of the jaw joint may occur and its movement is less full than it ought to be. Treatment of all these symptoms is possible once the condition is recognized.

Once the diagnosis is made and other causes of pain in the temporo-mandibular joint (jaw joint) such as arthritis have been excluded the trouble can be dealt with by a dental surgeon. Acute symptoms may require splinting of the joint for a short while to give relief. Where there is malocclusion of the teeth or where missing teeth hamper smooth closure of the jaw, the dental surgeon may have to do some reconstruction. Most patients who have been suffering from head pain secondary to jaw trouble benefit from exercises aimed at inducing relaxation of the affected muscle.

HEADACHE AND EXERCISE

"As for bodily exercises they must be used with discretion, neither are they to be practised of all men alike".

Thomas a Kempis

As far as exercise is concerned there are two groups — the believers and the non-believers! We might aptly divide them into the joggers and the non-joggers of our western world today. But if we extend the term exercise to include not only exercise deliberately undertaken, but any form of physical exertion, then we can consider how this relates to the subject of headache.

Any migraine sufferer knows how much worse the pain becomes when any physical effort is made during an attack. In a severe attack even raising the head from the pillow, or coughing, will intensify the pain. Many migraine sufferers have discovered from experience that strenuous physical effort can sometimes precipitate an attack. This is more often the case when other factors which contribute to the chain of events culminating in a migraine attack are also operating. Thus stress and hunger also have to be considered as possible important contributory factors when we think about exercise and headache.

During severe exercise the amount of blood pumped out by the heart per minute may rise to three times its resting value. The output of the heart per unit time is termed the cardiac output. The heart is made up of four compartments or chambers. Blood returns from the lungs and the rest of the body to the two auricles, and is pumped out to the lungs and the rest of the body from the ventricles of the heart. The stroke volume is the amount pumped out of each ventricle per beat and is about 80 ml. in a resting man of average size. The beats of the heart are felt in the pulse and if we assume that the average pulse rate is 70 beats per minute then we have a cardiac output of 80 × 70 ml. per minute which is 5.6 liters per minute. The output from the heart in a person lying quietly is the same as that during sleep, but the output can double with anxiety or excitement, and can rise sevenfold during very heavy physical exercise. The interesting fact is that although this increase in heart output has an affect throughout the body the blood flow to the brain remains remarkably constant at 750 ml/minute. In contrast to this the blood flow through exercising muscle may increase thirty-fold.

In the section of this book on the biochemistry of migraine the subject of vasoactive amines is dealt with in some detail. Amines are breakdown products of proteins and vasoactive amines are those which can affect the size of blood vessels. The chief of these vasoactive amines are the catecholamines, adrenaline and noradrenaline. The main breakdown product of the catecholamines is a substance called vanilmandelic acid and the excretion of this in the urine is increased not only under conditions of stress but also during and after exercise, particularly when the exercise is competitive in nature. In the latter circumstances there is also a measurable rise in the noradrenaline levels in the blood. These changes are closely connected with the biochemical changes resulting in headaches of the vascular type.

Tension headache is obviously likely to occur in conjunction with any sort of exercise which places a mental as well as a physical strain on a person liable to suffer from tension headaches.

During heavy exercise some people occasionally develop a dull, throbbing headache or may feel faint or giddy. When strenuous physical activity is undertaken there is a greatly increased demand for glucose in the muscles. Muscles store glucose in the form of glycogen, and when the blood sugar falls, as it does during fasting or exercise, this glycogen is rapidly mobilized and changed back into glucose. The catecholamines are released in response to a fall in blood sugar as they assist in the mobilization of glucose stores. It also seems probable that the nerves which control the size of the blood vessels are influenced by changes in blood sugar levels. When headaches frequently occur in association with extra exertion, be it cross country running or digging the garden, it is worth trying the effect of taking a drink sweetened with glucose before embarking on the exertion.

HEADACHE AND WORK

It is said of Maximilian II, King of Bavaria, who was born in 1811 and died in 1864, that he was a zealous, humorless, headache-prone scholarly man who would have preferred a professorship to being a king. He had two sons, Ludwig and Otto. Ludwig succeeded him as King and almost ruined his country by his building projects. The magnificant dream castles of Chiemsee, Neuschwanstein and Linderhof remain a memorial to him and a major attraction for tourists. Ludwig died by drowning, together with his doctor, in the Starnberger lake. The question is, however, might his father have been less headache prone had he been a professor and not a king?

When they first visit a doctor for any complaint patients are always asked about their occupation. This is not mere curiosity on the doctor's part, interesting though it may be to learn how other people earn their living. The work that we do can have a very real bearing on the symptoms that we develop and the way in which these symptoms respond to treatment. A driver, on shift work, for example, may find it a great deal more difficult to arrange the small regular meals needed in the treatment of a peptic ulcer than would a bank clerk working in one building, with regular hours.

Various occupational hazards are well recognized but since our subject is headache, we are concerned with whether there are certain occupations which make the people working in them particularly headache prone. There are some extremely rare causes of severe headache in relation to occupation. Thus workers in the meat industry occasionally develop Q fever. This is an infection in which the patient develops a high temperature and severe headache and often also an inflammation of the lungs. There are a number of substances that can be inhaled or ingested during the course of a working day and give rise to headache. The most obvious one is alcohol. Munitions workers sometimes complain of headaches which are due to changes in the size of their blood vessels following the inhalation of nitrites used in their work. Nitrites are of course prescribed in medical therapy to relieve the pain due to the constriction of blood vessels, such as anginal pain. Painters and sprayers not infrequently use paints and sprays containing headache-producing substances and the wearing of special masks may go a long way to relieving the symptoms. Mechanics and garage workers often work in poorly ventilated areas and develop the throbbing headache associated with carbon monoxide poisoning. Lead is another toxic substance which can give rise to headaches.

Stress is the most common cause of headache. Undoubtedly some occupations are more stressful than others. If we look around we can see that as well as having an amusing side to it there is a certain amount of truth in the Peter principle. This principle states that people often continue to be promoted up the ladder of their particular career until they reach the level at which they become incompetent. They stick at this level, but now life has become a strain and work is a burden. Few of us are wise enough to know how to be content before we reach this level — and whether the level is fairly near the bottom of the ladder or right at the top is immaterial. The effect will be the same.

The important fact to recognize is that our mental reactions to circumstances and situations have an effect on our body biochemistry. It is, for example, interesting that while we may willingly expend our energy on the tennis court or in cross country running when we enjoy these activities and may feel exhilirated and even refreshed by our achievements, many of us would complain of complete exhaustion if we were asked to put half the energy that we expend during a day's holiday into our daily work.

Hard work alone never did anyone any harm as long as those who work hard physically are fit and in training, and that those who work hard mentally are not finding it a strain. It is not what we do, but the way in which we react to the demands made upon us that is important. One of the hardest working members of any community is the mother who looks after several young children. The refrain of the Victorian Nannies' song was written for her:

"Long, long days, dear, and short, short nights".

Washing, ironing, cooking, feeding, she is constantly in demand for twenty four hours a day. But her work is a labor of love and in the words of Thomas a Kempis:

"Love feels no burden, thinks nothing of trouble, attempts what is above its strength, pleads no excuse of impossibility; for it thinks all things lawful for itself and all things possible.

It is therefore able to undertake all things, and it completes many things, and warrants them to take effect, where he who does not love, would faint and lie down."

Migraine sufferers sometimes report that they have managed to get through a time of severe strain with fewer headaches than usual. They may have been nursing a sick child or an elderly parent but a sense of duty or devotion has substained them and they have managed to meet the need. It suggests that our attitude to our problems is an important factor in how these problems affect us both mentally and physically.

When we exclude occupations in which there are clear links with headache precipitating factors we are left considering occupations in which the stresses and strains are such that they are likely to be the cause of headache. This, of course, depends largely on individual temperament. One person may find it an intolerable strain to work constantly within a tight time schedule, while another may find this precisely the challenge he enjoys in his daily work. Poring over figures all day may give one man a headache while another derives great satisfaction from completing painstaking, difficult work with accuracy. One cannot lay down rules about the type of work to which any individual is best suited. This depends on so many individual factors. What one can say, however, is that where any occupation becomes a daily source of anxiety and strain, it is worth giving the matter careful thought and looking into the possibility of change. The occurrence of headaches may act as a sign which indicates that thought along these lines is necessary.

HEADACHE AND HEAD INJURY

Undoubtedly headaches sometimes follow head injuries. Most of us have given our heads a hard knock at one time or another and would have been surprised had this not been followed by at least a temporary pain. This usually passes off fairly quickly and more persistent or recurring pain is rare. Sometimes patients who have had a head injury suffer from a brief loss of consciousness. This is called concussion, and may be followed by headache.

Various types of post traumatic headache have been reported. These are probably related to the part of the head that was damaged. When an artery has been involved short bursts of localized headache may occur. These may last for a short period, possibly only a few minutes of intense throbbing pain in the affected area. When a vein is damaged in the injury, pain may follow physical strain or exertion such as lifting a heavy suitcase. When a nerve has been affected painful spells may occur in a sharply defined area where the nerve carrying the pain fibres is pinched in the soft tissue. Children sometimes complain of pain in the back of the head for this reason. The "whiplash" type of injury may result in strain in the head and neck muscles resulting in pain.

Headaches following head injury usually clear up within three to six months.

Headaches after head injuries are more common in people who have a family history of migraine. This is not surprising as migraine in any case occurs significantly more frequently in people with a family history of migraine. Since migraine is a disorder of blood vessels, investigators have been interested in the possibility of changes in blood vessels occurring after head injuries.

Investigators have shown that after a severe head injury the blood vessels in the affected area may constrict. However, this spasm is only temporary so it does not look as if we can blame any attacks of migraine which occur after injury on any changes in the blood vessels resulting from the injury.

In recent years there have been a number of reports in the medical journals of typical attacks of migraine occurring for the first time, in close association with blows on the head, These attacks have occurred sufficiently often for the term "footballers migraine" to be coined; although of course they can arise just as readily in boxers, or in fact, following any sort of blow to the head. There have also been occasional reports of children suffering from a variety of neurological symptoms, such as transient paralysis, speech difficulty, giddiness and loss of balance following a blow to the head. These symptoms have lasted from a few minutes to several hours and have been associated with headache of varying severity and often also vomiting. They invariably clear up completely but at the time they closely resemble attacks of a severe type of migraine in which neurological symptoms are associated with head pain, nausea and vomiting. This type of headache and its possible mechanism is dealt with more fully in the section of this book dealing with migraine.

One has to remember that as with the symptoms following any injury to any part of the body, there is always a psychological factor. If you expect trouble you will probably find it.

Subdural Hematoma

A hematoma is a large blood clot. The fact that the brain is wrapped in three tissue-paper-like sheaths or envelopes was mentioned in the section of this book describing the skull and its contents. The outermost sheath is called the dura mater. In the chapter on the blood supply of the head one of the branches of the external carotid artery, called the middle meningeal, is mentioned. This runs from the outside of the skull, through a small hole called the foramen spinosum into the inside of the head, just within the dura mater. The course of the middle meningeal artery is on the side of the head and therefore in a vulnerable position as far as likely blows to the head are concerned. On rare occasions this vessel is damaged and starts to bleed. In the young the damage may be caused by a direct blow in sport or an accident. In the elderly the damage can follow a fall and be almost unsuspected. In any event, the development within the skull of a hematoma or blood clot occurs around the vessel. This presses on the underlying brain tissue and causes characteristic symptoms in which transient attacks of loss of consciousness or brief attacks of confusion can occur. Immediate surgical treatment is vital.

HEADACHE AND DEPRESSION

The author of the Old Testament book of Job is unknown, but the book was probably written roughly two and a half thousand years ago. Job was once a happy man of considerable wealth and influence who lived surrounded by a large and loving family. His fortunes, however, became drastically reversed and the book is a dialogue, first between Job and his friends and then between Job and Almighty God. Job's friends attempt to convince him that the miseries heaped upon him have arisen through his own fault and that he deserves his sorrows. Job knows this to be untrue. Not only has he lost the children he loved and the possessions that he worked for but he is inflicted with severe chronic illness. Job's attempts to understand the injustice of human sufering are expressed in words of exquisite poetry. Refuting the criticisms of his friends he finally puts his case to his Creator. Slowly Job comes to realize that God's ways are beyond human comprehension and in his realization he eventually finds peace.

Reflecting on his pain-filled days and sleepless nights Job spoke to his would be comforters:

"Is not man's life on earth nothing more than pressed
service, his time no better than hired drudgery?
Like the slave, sighing for the shade, or the workman
with no thought but his wages,
months of delusion I have assigned me,
nothing for my own but nights of grief.
Lying in bed I wonder "when will it be day"?
Risen I think, "How slowly evening comes"
Restlessly I fret till twilight falls."

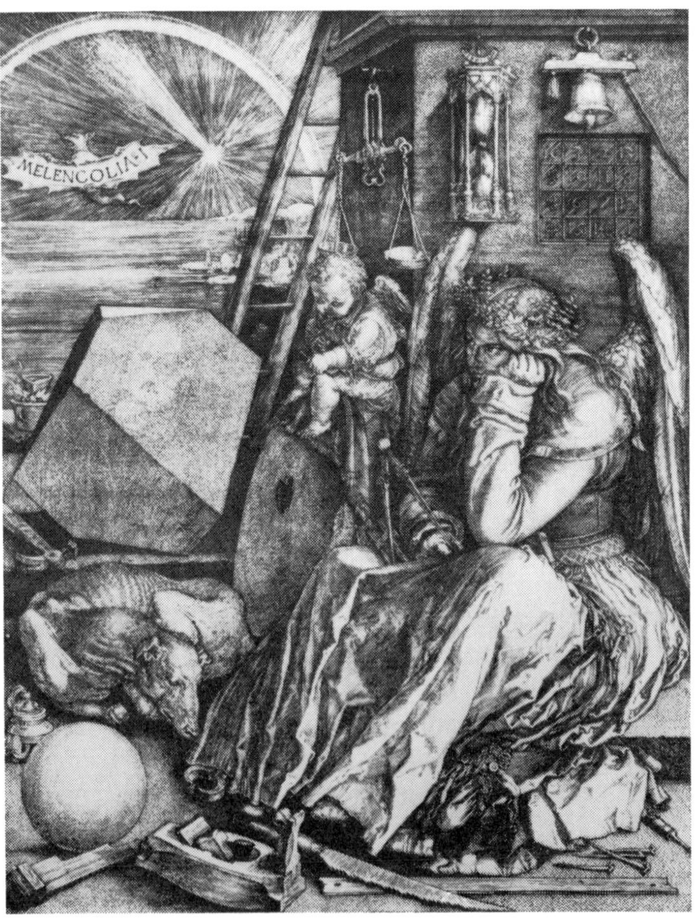

Engraving by Albrecht Durer.

Sufferers from tension headache who are also suffering from depression may see themselves reflected in the description of those who waken early in the morning and lie in bed worrying not only about "when will be it day" but also about the misfortunes which the coming day could bring. Migraine attacks often begin in the early hours of the morning and many a sufferer has spent the day in thinking

"How slowly evening comes"

Both tension headache and migraine sufferers will sympathise with Job's complaint

"Restlessly I fret till twilight falls".

It was not the loss of his worldly possessions that defeated Job. He was able to rise above this material blow. It was not the loss of his family. He was able to accept that what the Lord has given the Lord can take away. It was unremitting physical affliction which reduced Job to despair.

Depression can be divided into two main groups, endogenous and exogenous. Endogenous depression arises without any obvious cause. This type of depression is as much an illness as pneumonia or meningitis and requires expert medical help. The more common type of depression is termed exogenous depression. External circumstances have led the sufferer to feel that life is not really worth living, and that he cannot cope with all the things that are operating against him. Very often, of course, there is plenty of reason for the depressed person's state of mind and any practical steps that could be taken to relieve the strain should be taken.

Depression is an understandably common symptom in patients suffering from chronic pain. Some headache sufferers come into this group of depressed patients. Many of them are worried in case they have something really serious wrong with them like a brain tumor. But despite their anxiety they cannot bring themselves to put this fear into words. If they realized how rare such things are they might be relieved and go to consult their doctor, who could put their minds at rest.

A great deal can be done to help any headache sufferers

who also feel that life is not worth living. The fact that one brings one's problems out into the open goes some way towards helping to sort them out. The more we are in contact with other people the more we come to realize that our own worries are not unique. The fact that someone else is also carrying a heavy burden does not make your own load any lighter, but at least it helps to prevent the wholly destructive emotion of self pity from creeping in.

Today there are a large number of effective drugs for the treatment of depression. They are there to be used when needed, just as antibiotics are available for bacterial infections. No depressed patient should suffer needlessly, as treatment is available.

This section began with some brief comments on the book of Job, and the way in which he wrestled with the problem of suffering. Job had the light of the Old Testament to live by. We are more fortunate. It is only in the New Testament that we can begin to find the answer to the problem.

HEADACHE AND TRAVEL

Why do headache sufferers so often have an attack at the beginning of a holiday or when they are making a journey? It is such a common story that it is worth considering the possible reasons. The occasion may have been planned for weeks and anticipated with increasing pleasure. Then the day arrives and is completely ruined as the first sign of a headache appears. By this time, of course, the journey may already have started and there is no escape to familiar surroundings. So what can be done to make a headache less likely?

It is worth thinking about the reasons why headaches so often occur at this time.

The most common cause of headache is stress. Stress in this context includes such states as anxiety, excitement, anger, pleasure, frustration and fear. When we go on holiday we experience the excitement of getting away from our daily routine. Even a day trip to the seaside or a Sunday afternoon outing may give the same feeling.

If we are leaving for a longer period then there is the anxiety of getting everything ready on time and this may include packing for several members of the family. It almost inevitably includes the frustration of being unable to find some item, which precisely because it is lost, now appears to be essential to our luggage!

We may be travelling alone, or in company, but in either case anxieties arise. These vary from worrying over whether we shall meet someone pleasant to talk to, to worrying about the various factions which inevitably arise when a number of people have to adapt to each other, at close quarters, especially when the very young or the very old are included in the party. Even a one day outing can give rise to considerable stress. Just think of a family outing to the seaside or a day on your own at the Sales!

Migraine sufferers, in particular, should take some additional factors into account when arranging a holiday. For example, a small proportion of women tend to get headaches around the time of menstruation. If this is the case, it is obviously worth trying to arrange a journey at some other time in the month. Some migraine sufferers have noticed that certain foods seem to give them a headache. The foods most frequently mentioned are chocolate, cheese and alcoholic drinks. Even those who rarely drink alcohol are likely to celebrate the fact that work is over for a while, on the night before a holiday. This will probably be followed by a late night rushing around to make sure that nothing is forgotten. Next morning, there may not be time for even a hurried breakfast, despite the fact that in some headache sufferers fasting is a recognized cause of attacks. And even the awareness of its possible ill effects may not prevent the hasty eating of a bar of chocolate!

So far, we have been thinking of adults, but a similar patern of behavior applies equally to children at the beginning of a holiday or journey. They should be kept quietly occupied and avoid eating a lot of sweets and chocolates before setting off.

Having accepted the fact that for a number of reasons the beginning of a holiday or journey is likely to be associated with a headache then steps can be taken to make an attack less probable. The secret lies in planning ahead. Ten days before you plan to leave, take a large sheet of paper and make a list of all the things that you must remember to do. Put them under headings such as Home, Children, Work, Packing, etc. and stick the sheet where you can easily see it. Tick off each item as you deal with it and jot down the extra things that occur to you. Include everything from making arrangements about the daily papers to packing the baby's favorite toy. Start well in advance in order to make sure that the week before you leave is as unhurried and peaceful as possible.

There will be a number of things that you cannot do until the last minute, but list these separately and work out roughly how long each of them will take. Then when the day arrives, work your way through them in a methodical manner, knowing that you have sufficient time to finish them without a rush. This advice may seem very obvious, but if we are honest with ourselves we know that we seldom follow it unless we make a positive effort to do so. If, despite this, you know from past experience that you are going to find it difficult to keep calm, then ask your doctor to help you.

He may be willing to prescribe a mild tranquilizer, such as Valium for you, which you can take during the few days prior to your holiday and during your journey and on the night that you are travelling. A substance like "Tranxene" has been found to be particularly helpful by a lot of migraine sufferers, but this is obviously something that you must discuss with and let your own doctor decide. If you are a migraine sufferer you may find it helpful to take two soluble aspirin tablets in water on the evening before leaving and repeat this on the morning of departure.

The object of the aspirin is not to treat an as yet non existent headache, but to prevent the changes in the blood which are associated with the onset of a migraine attack from occurring. Having done all that you can to ensure an unruffled departure, then make sure that you leave yourself plenty of time for the journey. If you are worrying all the way to the air or sea port or the station about whether or not you will catch the boat, plane or train you will obviously undo all your earlier good work. Travel itself is often associated with sickness and headaches especially in children. Anyone who tends to suffer from travel sickness usually feels better in the front seat of the car or facing the engine of the train. Here your own doctor can help you by giving you a prescription for some anti-travel sickness tablets to take for the occasion.

If despite all these measures you feel the start of a headache, then act immediately. Do not wait to see whether or not it is going to develop. This is not a time for waiting to see. Take at once whatever treatment you usually find most help to you. Again you can ask your doctor to provide this before you leave.

As far as even more practical measures are concerned it is a wise precaution to take a supply of suitably sized strong polylthene bags on your journey. If you are going by car there is no problem as you can take a polylthene basin, but either bag or basin may lessen the acute misery of the headache sufferer who actually vomits while travelling.

And what about the holiday itself? It seems obvious that if you are unwise enough to totally change your habits, perhaps stay up very late at night, indulge in violent unaccustomed exercise and drink chianti by the bottle, it will hardly be surprising if you return from your holiday with a mournful tale of how your headaches prevented you from really enjoying yourself.

Meeting new people, adapting to strange circumstances, eating different food and engaging in fresh activities are all part of the average holiday. Unfortunately, however pleasant they may be, they are all a cause of stress. The only way to counteract this is by an attitude of mind. You have to decide right at the beginning of your holiday that you will do all you can to prevent your enjoyment being marred by headache symptoms and through understanding the causes of headaches you realize that these are partly under your control, and that you are able to help yourself very considerably.

HEADACHE AND WEATHER

The Sirocco winds are abnormally dry and hazy, bringing oppressive air from the hot desert interior of northern Africa to the Mediterranean. We read in the Old Testament that when Job had spoken from the depths of despair, one of his friends and would be comforters admonished him, saying "This is not a wise man's way, to answer with windy sophistries, as if thou hadst the Sirocco in thy blood . . . ." Most of us would agree that the weather influences how we feel. You have only to compare the difference between waking on a dull, grey damp day to wakening with the sunlight streaming through the windows. But can we blame changes in the weather for our headaches? Many people are convinced that they can and will tell you that they always know when it is going to thunder or rain because they always get a headache then. But is there any real proof that headaches can be linked with changes in the weather?

A carefully conducted investigation was carried out in London in an effort to discover whether or not there is an association between different types of weather and the occurrence of headache. Atmospheric conditions were recorded over a period of months in the year 1976 and at the same time a group of 310 patients attending the Princess Margaret Migraine Clinic for the treatment of an acute attack of headache were studied. The headache symptoms were then correlated with weather conditions. The Meteorological Office kindly supplied 3 hourly readings of barometric pressure, wind velocity, wind direction, temperature and humidity. The onset of headache was correlated with the weather conditions at that time and in some cases, with the weather readings 3 and 12 hours before the onset of headache attacks. A report on this work was produced by Dr. Marcia Wilkinson and Nurse Jane Woodrow and this concluded

"In the United Kingdom the variability of the barometric pressure is so small that it does not appear to have any influence on the incidence of headache. The prevailing winds in Britain are from the south-west and north-east and most headaches occurred when the winds were in these directions. Tension headaches tend to occur with higher wind velocity but this seems to make no difference in the onset of migraine attacks. A drop in temperature and a rise in humidity 3 hours before the onset of headache appears to be of some significance.

Of the patients attending the Clinic for treatment of an acute attack 60% developed their headaches between 6 and 9 a.m. and 1.5% between 9 p.m. and 3 a.m. while in the group of 100 non-acute patients 39% developed headaches between 6 and 9 a.m. and 5% developed headaches between 9 p.m. and 5 a.m."

As the report on this London study pointed out one has to remember that the weather in Britain is not subject to the extreme variations in climate that occur in other parts of the world. Similar studies to those in London were undertaken in the University of Uppsala in Sweden where Professor P.O. Lundberg reported —

"The effect of changes in some weather and indoor climate parameters on headache was studied in 60 healthy persons working in two different types of buildings during a two months period in the autumn. Self-registration of headache days and headache index were used. Headache data were calculated for a working day and the day after a working day.

Daily weather observations (temperature, precipitation, wind, air-pressure, cloudiness) at 7.00 a.m. were obtained from the Department of Meteorology. A subjective weather index was also used. The atmospheric ratio noise at 27 kc/s was continuously recorded. Sound and infrasound levels were registered at calm and windy periods.

The electrostatic charging of each individual was measured with an electrostatic voltmeter. As further indoor climate parameters small positive and negative air ions as well as the concentration of small particles in the air were measured for 17 different days in each of the two buildings. Temperature and relative humidity were also continuously recorded.

To study any time delay of the influence from the assumed initiating factors cross covariance functions of headache data and each of the physical parameters were calculated for zero up to seven days.

The most interesting finding was a peak incidence or more headache on "bad" weather days. There was also a clear tendency for more headaches on the day before windy weather. No significant influence of static electricity, air ions or air particles on headache was found."

Winds, in particular, have been blamed for symptoms of ill health. For example, headaches, irritability, and an increase in respiratory ailments have been attributed to the Foehn. The Foehn is a warm, relaxing wind experienced on the leeward or northern side of the Alpine range in Europe. It occurs most frequently in winter and early spring but can blow at all seasons. During its descent from the mountain slopes the wind changes in character from being cool and moist to dry and warm.

Foehn-like weather is characterized by three features. Not only is it dry and warm but the relative humidity of the atmosphere falls and the temperature rises 5 to 10 °C above the average for the time of year. The third feature is that the presence of hot, dry air currents is preceded by a high level of positive ions.

In Israel, the hot dry winds are called Sharav. Dr. F.G. Sulman of the Department of Pharmacology in the Hebrew University of Jerusalem has studied patients who complain of what he calls the "Irritation Syndrome" during the time of the Sharav. This irritation syndrome manifests itself by a wide variety of symptoms, such as irritability, sleeplessness, allergic complaints and flushes, but the one in which we are particularly interested is headache. Dr. Sulman[1] investigated biochemical changes in 200 patients suffering from Sharav. He measured a number of biochemical parameters in these patients but the most striking finding was that in the day or two prior to Sharav, a greatly increased excretion of 5-hydroxytryptamine and its breakdown product 5-hydroxyindole acetic acid was found in the urine of individuals suffering from the irritation syndrome. The finding is highly relevant to the biochemical changes known to occur in migraine attacks. These changes are described in the section of this book on the biochemistry of migraine. 5-hydroxytryptamine is a substance which can have a powerful effect on blood vessels. The levels of 5-hydroxytryptamine in the blood rise sharply prior to the onset of a migraine attack. One of the chief break-down products of 5-hydroxytryptamine is 5-hydroxyindole acetic acid and the levels of this in the urine rise during an attack of migraine. Thus the findings of changes in 5-hydroxytryptamine metabolism in relation

---

[1]Proceedings of the International Headache Symposium, Elsinore, Denmark, 16-18 May 1971, p. 205.

to the incidence of headaches must be taken seriously in relation to the incidence of headaches. It is also of interest that the patients who suffered from the Sharav irritation syndrome benefitted from the use of drugs which counteract the effects of 5-hydroxytryptamine.

However, while this report from Israel will please those who are convinced that climate can influence their headache symptoms, this is still an area in which it is so easy to be prejudiced that scepticism is wise until the whole subject has been investigated more fully.

HEADACHE AND SMOKING

Some headache sufferers are convinced that being in a smoky atmosphere gives them a headache. This may well be true. If you dislike smoking and the clinging smell of tobacco in your clothes, and feel sufficiently strongly about it, there is little doubt that a tension headache could result. But there may be more to it than this. Apparently nicotine can increase the output of catecholamines in the blood and the section of this book dealing with migraine explains how catecholamines are concerned in the production of a migraine attack. Similarly, research into factors concerned with the aggregation of small particles in the blood called platelets indicates that these may clump together or aggregate more readily under the influence of smoking.

The headache sufferers who associate some of their headaches with smoking are probably fortunate. At least it makes them less likely candidates for lung cancer and coronary thrombosis!

HEADACHE AND SLEEP

Sleep overcomes us in the absence of physical or mental stimulation. This is why people choose a quiet, darkened room when they want to sleep. It also explains why we all know the torture of keeping awake during a boring discussion. On many occasions, only the thought of the unfortunate guest at a meeting, who not only nodded off but toppled off his chair on the platform into the first row of the audience in front of him, has kept me awake! All living creatures have regular periods when they rest and become unaware of their surroundings.

The section of this book dealing with epilepsy mentions E.E.G. changes and rapid eye movements (R.E.M.). During sleep there are alternate phases of R.E.M. sleep alternating with non R.E.M. and slow wave sleep. R.E.M. sleep occupies about 20% of total sleep time and is associated with dreaming and an increased blood supply to the brain.

Sleep is necessary to us. It is part of the circadian or twenty-four hour rhythm of our bodies. Certain changes occur during sleep. Our kidneys secrete a more concentrated urine and its volume falls. The level of catecholamine

181

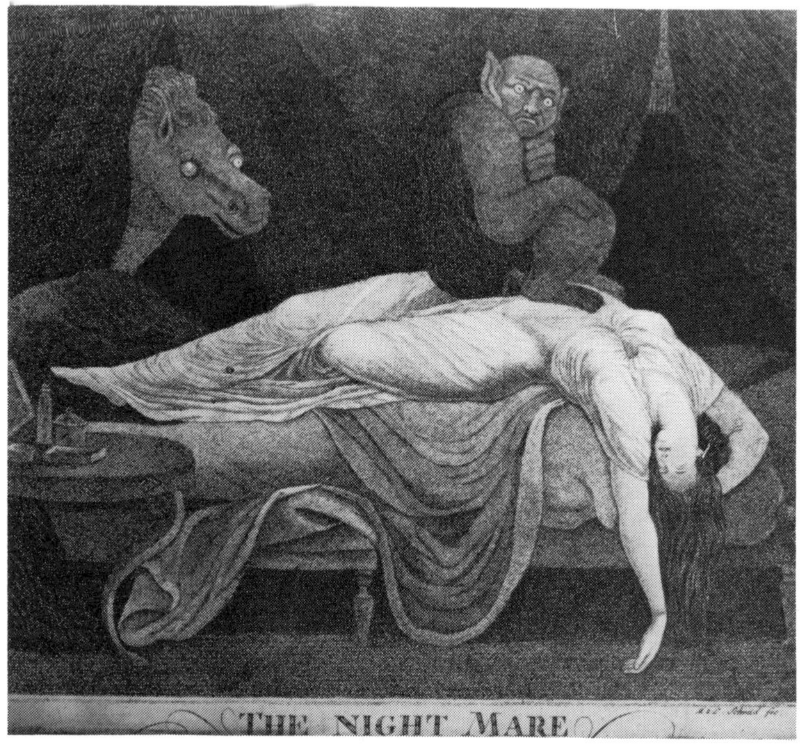

excretion falls to its lowest levels during the early hours of each new day and the tone of our blood vessels changes during sleep.

It is of interest that research in patients who sometimes wake in the early hours of the morning with an attack of migraine has revealed a sharp rise in catecholamine levels in the blood prior to the onset of headache. R.E.M. sleep is also reported to precede waking with an attack.

Knowing that moderation in all things should be the motto of any headache sufferer no-one will be surprised to learn that both too little or too much sleep can be causes of headache. One or two late nights may be enough to precipitate a headache. Similarly the luxury of an extra hour or two in bed in the morning may lead to a throbbing headache on waking. This is particularly the case with migraine sufferers. Sometimes one or two extra pillows are helpful in preventing this especially if these are put under the head at the usual time of waking. A light warm shawl around the head can be helpful. After all, the rest of the body is kept warm in bed and only the head is exposed. Many people like to sleep with open windows and howling gales are not unknown in bedrooms. Vascular tone changes with temperature and we know that changes in vascular tone are sometimes associated with the onset of headache. Whatever the merits of keeping a cool head in the decisions of life may be, a comfortably warm head is a good insurance as far as headache is concerned.

PAIN

"There screened in shades from days detested glare
Spleen sighs for ever on her pensive bed
Pain at her side and megrim at her head."

Alexander Pope (1688—1744)

A naturally occurring pain killer, called enkephalin, was isolated from brain tissue in 1975. This exciting discovery has provided an enormous stimulus to research into pain and how it is produced. Enkephalin acts like morphine. The chief drawback to the use of morphine is the fact that it is an addictive drug. Unfortunately when enkephalin is prevented from breaking down naturally, as it does in brain tissue, it too becomes addictive. However, since enkephalin was identified other molecules of the same family, known as endorphins, have been found and it is hoped that further research will reveal a satisfactory substitute for morphine. In any event, more work in this area is bound to increase our understanding of the nature of pain and its relief.

The word pain is derived from the Latin word "poena." The Latin word is translated as penalty or retribution and in primitive societies pain was often regarded as a punishment from the gods. Pain is usually associated with inflammation. The classical description of inflammation was given by Celsus, a Roman nobleman, who lived at the time of Christ. Celsus was a follower of Hippocrates the father of medicine and he wrote books on philosophy, military science, agriculture, law and medicine. Only the book on medicine, first printed in Florence in 1476, is still in existence. Celsus describes inflammation by four signs, calor, rubor, tumor, dolor — heat, readness, swelling and pain.

Pain serves a protective function by indicating that something is amiss. In a rare neurological disorder, called syringomyelia, the sense of pain is lost. Patients suffering from this illness no longer have an inbuilt warning system and because they have no feeling they knock and burn and injure their fingers and toes which then easily become ulcerated and infected.

Pain is transmitted through the nerve endings in the skin and internal organs. The causes and types of pain differ in different parts of the body. For example, your lungs distend with air with every breath and this is painless but severe flatulence can be very painful. The muscles of the limbs contract without pain but contractions of uterine muscle can produce pain.

The pain threshold is the level at which pain is felt. This varies from one person to another. If a person is in good health and feels fit he is able to tolerate pain better than a person who is tired, overanxious and run down. On the whole children have a higher pain threshold than adults. A method has been found for measuring the pain threshold and one can see how this threshold differs between one person and another. One way of measuring the pain threshold of a person is by applying pressure with a thin tube over the mastoid process or bump just behind the lobe of the ear. The pressure required to produce the beginnings of a painful sensation varies from half a kilogram to six kilograms per square centimeter, but the majority of people feel pain with a pressure of about two kilograms. Surprisingly enough, women tend to feel pain at a lower threshold than men.

A lot of interesting work has been done in attempts to discover how pain is produced and why it occurs. In some of this research a cantharidin plaster has been applied to a small area of smooth skin such as the forearm, about one centimeter in diameter. The plaster is left on overnight and by the next morning a blister will have formed. The fluid in this blister is gently sucked out with a small needle and syringe and the dead skin of the blister is carefully cut away. This leaves the raw area at the blister exposed. Normal saline, which is salt solution made up to the same strength as the salt solution contained in the blood, causes no pain when applied to this raw area. The area is, however, highly sensitive to chemical irritants. If the blister fluid which was sucked out of the blister is kept in a glass tube for an hour and then dropped back on to the raw blister severe pain results. Why should this occur when the fluid previously protected the raw area and caused no pain? The interesting fact is that during the hour that the blister fluid was kept in the glass tube a substance developed in the blister fluid and this is responsible for producing the severe pain when the fluid is reapplied. The blister fluid consists of plasma containing protein. Contact with glass activates this protein and breaks it down. A pain producing substance called bradykinin is produced. Normal blood consists of red blood cells, white blood cells and the fluid plasma. Plasma contains a group of substances called kinins and these are associated with the production of pain. The best known kinins are bradykinin and kallidin. If pure bradykinin is applied to the blister base, even in minute concentrations it can provoke pain. The pain produced by bradykinin usually rises gradually to a peak which is maintained for a time before subsiding. It also produces pain when it is injected under intact skin or into an artery. When a minute dose is injected into the carotid artery it produces severe pain along the branches of the external carotid artery but the effect differs with the dosage used. At one dosage level intense pain occurs in the head with perhaps temporary partial loss of vision and nausea. If the dose is only one fifth as large, the vessels in the affected area simply dilate and become more permeable.

An increase in vascular permeability is characteristic of pain production and is common to all types of inflammation, whether it occurs in the joints as in rheumatoid arthritis or in the head as in migraine. Permeability implies that vessels allow substances that are normally contained in them to diffuse through into the surrounding tissues. In the section of this book dealing with the biochemistry of migraine, a substance called 5-hydroxytryptamine (5HT) has been frequently mentioned. 5HT is thought to be one of the main mediators of tissue permeability and is closely concerned with pain production. Another group of substances probably concerned in pain production are prostaglandins. They are fatty substances which have a marked effect on blood vessels, and are known to be involved in many different types of acute and chronic inflammatory processes producing pain. An intravenous infusion of one type of prostaglandin, prostaglandin E_1, can cause severe headache. Aspirin and certain other pain relieving substances often used in the treatment of headache are known to inhibit the production of prostaglandins.

And now we return to the recent discovery of endorphins with which this selection on pain began. May their discovery fulfill the promise which they appear to offer to pain research.

HEADACHES AND HOMOEOPATHY

*"Hahnemann's physiognomy contains all the indica-
tions of a remarkable and self confident intelligence,
an unbending will and an undaunted energy.*

*He was too ambitious to lose himself in dreams; he
was too self-willed and stubborn to tread the beaten
track. If he followed a tradition it must be one that
was eternal; when he expounded a teaching he could
tolerate denial but not discussion."*

*from L'Homoeopathie Francais
Revue Mensuelle. 1912. No.1*

Samuel Hahnemann was a remarkable man. Born in
Meissen, in Germany, in 1755 he studied medicine but
became a rebel against the orthodox practice of his day. In
1790 when he was translating Dr. William Cullens
"Materia Medica" he was struck by the fact that the most
successful drug for any condition appeared to be that
which itself produced toxic symptoms similar to those being treated. It was the actions of quinine which first drew
Hahnemann to make this observation which had already
been recorded many centuries earlier. More than 500 years
before the Birth of Christ Hippocrates stated that drugs
could sometimes cure "similar" diseases.

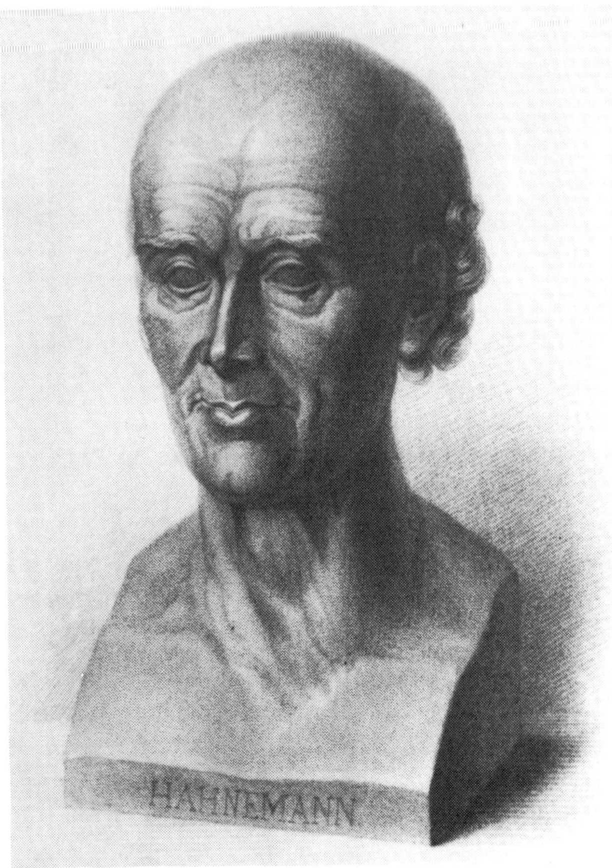

Samuel Hahnemann

Two thousand years after Hippocrates, Samuel Hahnemann became the founder of homoeopathy. Homoeopathic treatment is based on the principle that what a substance can cause it can also cure. The homoeopath uses minute quantities of drugs, which are obtained from plants, salts, metals and venoms. The actual substances are often the same as those used in conventional medical practice but the homoeopath uses them in very much smaller doses and the conditions in which they are employed may be different. For example, atropine is one of the alkaloids contained in belladonna which occurs naturally in the berry of deadly nightshade. Atropine dries up secretions and produces dilated pupils, a flushed face and a dry mouth. It is used every day in conventional medical practice in the injections given to patients about to have an operation because it has been found that the incidence of post-operative pneumonia is greatly reduced when the lungs are "dry" during anaesthesia. The homoeopath uses belladonna for disorders in which the face is flushed, the mouth dry and the pupil dilated. For example, Dr. Hahnemann believed that belladonna had a particular protective action in epidemics of scarlet fever, where the bright flushed face and hot dry skin call to mind the toxic effects of belladonna.

Thus the homoeopath treats symptoms rather than diseases. If a disease presents a number of symptoms such as headache, nausea, joint pain and colic the homoeopathic practitioner will first select the dominant symptom and treat this with minute doses of a substance, which, if taken in larger amounts, would produce the same symptom. Homoeopaths prefer to prescribe only one drug at a time. At least homoeopathic therapy is unlikely to cause iatrogenic disease. This is disease resulting from drug therapy and sometimes arises from our conventional therapy, and large dosage of a number of different drugs.

Blood letting or bleeding was a standard practice for the treatment of many diseases in Hahnemann's day. He opposed this bitterly and this opposition alone probably led to the saving of countless lives particularly during the cholera epidemic which swept across Europe from Eastern Russia in 1831.

In the treatment of headache homeopathic therapy is directed at very carefully assessed symptoms. Thus a throbbing, burning headache which is periodic in occurrence and accompanied by anxiety and restlessness, and in which the pain is aggravated by movement and the head tender to touch, is treated with minute doses of arsenic. The headache that is treated with bryony is a severe pain, dull and throbbing with acute sharp stabbing pains at intervals, especially after movement. The type of headache treated by the homoeopath with bryony is felt largely over the eyes and relieved by pressure and cool poultices.

The treatment of headache with Gelsemium is also mentioned in the homoeopathic materia medica [1]. Gelsemium is a drug obtained from the dried root of the plant Gelsemium semper virens. This used to be used in tincture form for the treatment of neuralgic pain. It is now little used in ordinary medical practice but in homoeopathic practice gelsemium is still recommended for the treatment of headache of sudden onset, often beginning with blurring of sight or double vision. The headache is usually worse in the morning. Sulphur is also said to affect the head in all regions, forehead, vertex and occiput, perhaps most characteristically the vertex. The headaches for which sulphur therapy is recommended are associated with flushes and often recur at intervals. The homoeopathic materia medica states "In spite of the general desire of sulphur patients for fresh air, the headaches (especially if one-sided sick headaches) are often worse in fresh air and relieved in a warm room. The head is hot and flushed and probably the brain congestion is relieved by the warm atmosphere that draws more blood to the surface. Exactly the opposite phenomenon is characteristic of arsenium where the headaches are relieved by fresh air, though the patient generally needs warmth and hates cold of any kind. With the pain goes the characteristic of burning . . .".

Again, in connection with headache sepia is mentioned. Sepia is a substance obtained from the ink bag of the cuttle fish, and ranks among the most important of homoeopathic remedies although it is unknown outside homoeopathic practice. It owes its presence in the Materia Medica to Dr. Hahnemann. The following passage is taken from the Materia Medica:

"The headaches associated with sepia are severe, hemicrania is common (with ocular symptoms, flashes of light and disturbed vision), the pains are violent and often throbbing . . . A good sleep relieves it, but if the patient is awakened from a short sleep the headache is aggravated. Such headaches are intensified by moving about the house, but vigorous exercise in the open air helps to work off the headache. Thundery weather makes the headache worse and is disturbing to the sepia patient in most ways. Vertigo may be accompanied by the sensation as of something 'rolling round' in the head . . . .".

It is clear from these brief extracts that the homoeopathic physician treats his headache sufferers on an entirely individual basis and does not resort to the use of the common analgesic drugs such as aspirin, paracetomol or codeine, which are so readily prescribed in our conventional medical practice. This very careful assessment of individual symptomatology is essential to homoeopathic practice, and one cannot doubt that this attention to detail alone would be of benefit in a number of disorders.

There were many, however, who failed to agree with the therapies prescribed and the therapeutic approach preached by Samuel Hahnemann. In his later years his personal life also gave rise to considerable criticism. After nearly 48 years of happy married life, during which she had borne him eleven children, his first wife died in 1830. At first his two youngest daughters took care of their widowed father, until, to their surprise, he embarked on a second marriage at the age of 80. His bride was a Frenchwoman, fifty years his junior, She had come from Paris, dressed as was sometimes the custom for young women travelling in that day, in boys clothing, to consult him. Within three months she had married him and shortly afterwards, in 1835, persuaded him to cut adrift from his family and accompany her back to Paris. Here she was active in promulgating his homoeopathic art both before and after his death in 1843. His final resting place, after his initial burial in the cemetery of Montmartre, is in the Pere Lachaise Cemetery in Paris. Here a monument to him now stands. Another monument to Dr. Hahnemann forms one of the outstanding sights of the American capital, Washington. This was unveiled at the turn of the century in an impressive ceremony at which President McKinley, a supporter of homoeopathy, was present. The founder of homoeopathy is seated on a mighty pedestal bearing the inscription which sums up his work:

"Similia simulibus".

(Like with like)

REFERENCES

1. An Introduction to the Principles and Practice of Homoeopathy. By Charles E. Wheeler. London. William Heinemann (Medical Books) Ltd., 1940.

UNUSUAL REMEDIES AND HEADACHE

"Weave a circle round him thrice,
And close your eyes with holy dread.
For he on honey-dew hath fed
And drunk the milk of Paradise".

Kubla Khan. S.T. Coleridge.

The fact that a number of unusual remedies exist or keep cropping up for the treatment of a disorder usually implies that no wholly satisfactory method of treatment, either orthodox or otherwise, is yet available. Nowhere is this more apparent than in the treatment of headache. Just as the sale of hope in a box has made vast fortunes for cosmetic manufacturers, so the hope of obtaining a cure will lure sufferers from all kinds of disorders to try any new and promising therapy. In the past few years a number of new treatments have received considerable publicity in the headache field and one of the most interesting is acupuncture.

ACUPUNCTURE

The subject of acupuncture has aroused increasing

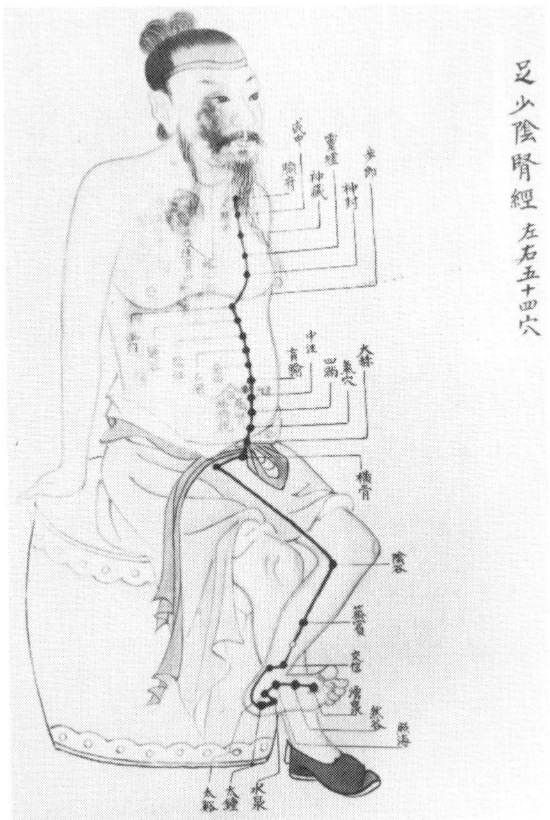

Chinese acupuncture chart.

interest in the West. Devised by the Chinese as a method of treatment many centuries of time. We do not understand how it works in the relief of pain and it puzzles and fascinates us as a method that is foreign to our way of thinking. Chinese medicine differs from our own because it is founded on ancient philosophical concepts. This is far removed from the mathematical logic and experimental observation on which our modern scientific medicine is based.

In the last twenty-five years the practice of acupuncture has increased in the Western world. It is used particularly in France and Germany. An International

Institute of Acupuncture has been formed and there is also a French Institute of Acupuncture. The subject of Acupuncture is recognized by the Faculty of Medicine in Paris.

Another term for acupuncture is needling, which tells us in one word what it is about. Acupuncture is performed by the use of needles. Traditionally these needles were of nine kinds, arrow headed, blunt, puncturing, spearpointed, ensiform, round, capillary, long and great. They were made of steel, copper or silver with brass wire handles. The needles were inserted into the flesh at depths and sites varying with the condition to be treated. Sometimes a light blow from a mallet was necessary in order to insert the needle. The needles were used either hot or cold. If heating was required then herbs were placed around the brass wire at the end of the needle and ignited. The needles were left in position for varying lengths of time. They might be left for a few minutes or for much longer periods, even up to days on end.

The technique of acupuncture was derived from the ancient Chinese philosophical concept of opposing forces in nature. Everything was related to the elements, the planets, the seasons and the time of day. Everything possessed the qualities of Yang and Yin in varying proportions. The idea of Yang was associated with light, the sun, the south and with maleness. The idea of Yin was associated with darkness, the moon, the north and femaleness. In order to lead a good life and to maintain health a perfect balance between Yang and Yin was necessary. If this balance was disturbed in a human being disease resulted and the method of acupuncture was devised as a means of restoring harmony between the opposing forces of Yin and Yang.

According to Chinese tradition the contrasting components Yin and Yang are carried in a series of separate channels in the human body. These channels are called meridians. Models of the human body showing these meridians and acupuncture points are made and date from ancient times. The acupuncture points lie either on the meridians or at their intersections. Traditionally there are 365 acupuncture points along twelve meridians. The site chosen for acupuncture is related only in an empirical way to the area in which pain is to be relieved. The time at which acupuncture may be performed in Chinese medicine is closely related to the seasons and time of the month. For example, on the third day of the month acupuncture of the thigh was forbidden. On the sixteenth day acupuncture of the chest was forbidden.

The functions of the body are controlled in two ways. They are under the control of chemical messengers called hormones. These are secreted into the bloodstream by a number of endocrine glands such as the pituitary gland and the thyroid gland and the concentration of the hormones in the bloodstream controls a variety of activities. The second way in which the actions of the body are controlled and co-ordinated is through the nervous system.

The nervous system consists of two parts. One of these is the central nervous system comprising the brain and spinal cord with the nerves arising from them. It receives sensory impulses and controls voluntary movement. The other, the autonomic nervous system, regulates those functions of which we are unaware and which are completely beyond our conscious control, such as the rate of the heart beat and the movement of the intestine. It is a highly complex system composed of two parts, the sympathetic and the parasympathetic. The actions of these two parts are opposite in effect, for example the sympathetic fibers dilate the pupil and cause an increase in the rate of the heart beat. Stimulation of the parasympathetic fibers constricts the pupils and slows the heart rate.

One of the main functions of the sympathetic nervous system is to control the size of the blood vessels. The actions of the autonomic nervous system are brought about by chemical means. There are two chemical transmitters in the autonomic nervous system, namely acetylcholine and noradrenaline. The chemical which is usually released at the ends of sympathetic nerve fibers is noradrenaline which, like adrenaline, belongs to a group of substances called catecholamines. The catecholamines are produced in the body in two ways. Under certain conditions they are secreted by the suprarenal glands, which are small glands situated just above the kidneys. They are also released at the ends of sympathetic nerve fibers where they supply organs such as blood vessels. When the catecholamines are released by the suprarenal glands they augment the effect of stimulation of the sympathetic nervous system.

When the two parts of the autonomic nervous system, the sympathetic and the parasympathetic systems were first described they were likened to the opposing forces of Yang and Yin. Acupuncture has been used chiefly in the treatment of such conditions as headache and arthritis.

This approach to therapy may seem strange to our Western minds but there is no doubt that acupuncture can be a successful method of relieving pain. The fact that we do not understand why or how this takes place does not alter the fact that it can be a highly successful therapy.

During the process of acupuncture, while the needles are in position, a constant stimulation of the tissues is undertaken. Either the needles are constantly twirled around by hand, or they are heated. Nowadays an electric current may be passed between two needles. The relief of pain or production of anaesthesia may develop very slowly. Anaesthesia sometimes lasts for several hours after the needles are withdrawn. The use of acupuncture as a means of inducing anaesthesia in surgery is of particular interest. The needles may be inserted at some distance from the site of operation. For example the removal of a stomach may be undertaken under anaesthesia produced by the insertion of four acupuncture needles in the lobes of the ear.

Acupuncture was one of the chief methods available to a Chinese physician. Confucius (551-479 B.C.) objected strongly to the dissection of the human body after death or any cutting of the body in life. Surgery, therefore, could not develop under the Chinese system.

Some sceptics dismiss acupuncture as a form of hypnosis or autosuggestion. Doubtless faith on the part of the patient plays an integral part in the success of the method and the Chinese belief in acupuncture is based on the tradition of many centuries. Only about one in five people respond to hypnotism and the success rate with acupuncture is considerably higher than this which leaves one wondering by what other means the technique of acupuncture produces its effects.

As far as the pain of migraine attacks is concerned it is a fact that one in four migraine sufferers is likely to benefit from almost any new therapy, at least for a while. One would therefore anticipate that if all migraine sufferers were given treatment by acupuncture about one quarter of them would report an improvement in their symptoms. It is difficult to see how one could ever undertake a controlled investigation into the efficacy of acupuncture in the treatment of headache but the facts will gradually have to speak for themselves as more sufferers try this method. This will take time, but we should be able gradually to collect and assess the evidence. At the same time, further investigations and new theories of pain may eventually explain why the method is so often successful.

AUTO-ACUPRESSURE

It is of interest that a "do it yourself at home" modification of acupuncture techniques has recently been given publicity. It is called auto-acupressure. The basis of this method of therapy is the application of pressure in a certain way on specific points in the body.

Just as a student of first aid learns how and where to apply pressure in order to deal with bleeding from different arterial sites, so the headache sufferer is taught how and where to apply pressure for different types of headache. Auto-acupressure is applied with the two thumbnails. The aim is to apply hard pressure on a small area through which the nerve supplying the painful site on the head passes. Auto-acupressure is a technique that has to be acquired with patience and practice.

YOGA

Yoga is another method of achieving control over bodily functions. Although we have come to associate it with a system of exercises undertaken in efforts to attain greater bodily fitness and relaxation, it was originally derived from Hindu philosophy. In this context attempts are made to divert the senses from the external world and to concentrate thought within. Both yoga and biofeedback techniques try to achieve the mastery of mind over matter, and any success in the treatment of headache is due to this.

FAITH HEALING

The fact that faith healers are sometimes very successful in treating certain types of headache symptoms should come as no surprise. The most common cause of headache is tension and it is obvious that sufficient faith may well help to relieve stress and strain. A fascinating example of faith healing is seen in Valentine Greatrakes who was born in Ireland in 1628. In a letter addressed to the Honourable Robert Boyle Esq. [1], he gives a brief account of the "divers and strange cures by him lately performed". He outlines his career which included service as an officer in Oliver Cromwell's army, followed by a period as Clerk of the Peace of the County of Cork, on which he comments "In which Employment I studied so to acquit myself before God and Man in singleness and integrity of heart, that to the comfort of my Soul and praise of Gode that directed me, I can with confidence say, I never took Bribe or Reward from any man, though I have had many and great ones offered me . . .".

Commenting on the religious intolerance of his day and on the way in which he had always tried to mete out justice to all men alike, he wrote "for that Charity had left Religion, which too many made a meer design to promote their Interests and Faction: thus one Faction destroyed another, till at length they all lay down in sorrow, and he that was most violent still came to the worst."

At that time the disease of scrofula was rife. Scrofula was the name given to a tuberculous inflammation of lymph glands in the neck which became enlarged and sometimes suppurated or discharged. Legend had it that the King's touch could cure scrofula and it became known as the King's evil. Greatrakes felt a growing conviction that he had been given the power of curing the King's evil by the laying on of hands. The first cure reported in a long letter to the Hon. Robert Boyle was of a child. Greatrakes wrote "... on which my wife told me there was one that had the Kings-Evil very grievously in the Eyes, Cheek and Throat; whereupon I told her that she should now see whether this were a bare fancy or imagination as she thought it, or the dictates of God's spirit on my heart; and thereupon I laid my hands on the places affected and prayed to God for Jesus sake to heal him, and then I bad the parent two or three days afterward to bring the child to me again, which accordingly he did, and then I saw the Eye was almost quite whole, and the Node, which was almost as big as a pullets egg, was suppurated, and the throat strangely amended, and to be brief (to Gods glory I speak it) within a month discharged it felt quite and was perfectly healed, and so continues God to be praised."

Valentine Greatrakes performed his healing by the laying on of hands combined with prayer and faith. Since we are especially interested in the healing of headache the following testimonials to his healing powers will be of particular interest. They are quoted in full in the letter addressed by Greatrakes to Robert Boyle.

Mr. Langhams Certificate

These are to certifie, That whereas I had been daily troubled with the Head-ach, more or less, for full three years together, hardly a day omitted, especially when after Riding I was most unsufferably tormented; I have by God's great blessing (ever since Mr. Valentine Greatrak's touched me in His Highness Prince Ruperts Chamber) been very well and free from anything of the Headach; and since my being stroked I have rid from Dover to London in ten hours. Given under my Hand and Seal, this 27th day of March, 1666.

I suppose from the time I received this benefit to this day above written, is full three weeks.

Thomas Langhame

Mrs. Smiths Certificate

Mary, Wife of Arthur Smith, a Mercer at the Lyon within Ludgate, aged 23, troubled with a great and continued pain in her forehead for the space of ten years, notwithstanding the use of the best Physicians and most excellent Remedies, to her Parents great Cost; about the latter end of March 1665/6 applied herself to Mr. Greatrak's, who laid his hand upon her Forehead, whereby the pain removed in to the hinder part of her head and neck, thence to the crown of her head, and from thence into her cheek, where it continued swelled, until she was again stroked in that part the day following; whereupon the swelling and pain vanished and never troubled her any more. Attested this first of May 1666.

Mary Smith

In presence of   Anne Meyrn

J. Fairclough, M.D.   Mother of the Party

It is interesting to speculate about the types of headache from which Thomas Langhame and Mary Smith were suffering. The fact that they were unremitting in character and that no other distinguishing features were mentioned suggest that they may have been severe tension headaches. Even those who find it hard to accept that enough faith could move mountains would not therefore be too surprised if patients with this type of headache were much improved by the attention of a physician in whom they had great trust. Valentine Greatrakes was less successful in his attempts to cure Lady Ann Finch Conway who suffered from the age of 12 until her death in 1678 at the age of 47 from such severe attacks of migraine that the great physician Thomas Willis wrote at the end of the treatise on her complaint

"For from any other cause, if there had been a conflict of Nature's medicine with the Disease, either a quick death or a foyful Victory had far sooner been attained."

Greatrakes himself died in the year 1683.

HYPNOTISM

Franz Anton Mesmer was born in Australia in 1734. He invented the method of treatment called mesmerism which was the forerunner of modern hypnotism. Mesmer believed that a force which he called animal magnetism permeated the universe and that there was a healing and magnetic power in his own hands. He studied medicine in Vienna, passing his final examinations in 1765. Like Paracelsus, a Swiss physician of the sixteenth century, Mesmer believed that human health can be influenced by the stars. When just 32 years of age he wrote a paper 'Disputatis de Planetarum Influxu" (Concerning the Influence of the Planets) which contained the germ of his theories. These were later stated in "Twenty Seven Propositions". Mesmer confined his healing activities to sufferers from disorders of the nervous system and made no secret of his method which he described as increasing the flow of magnetism in the body. Thus his instructions to his pupils are given here, and it is of particular interest that the disorders for which the therapy is used include the cure of violent headache. Mesmer's instructions were as follows:—

You must place yourself opposite to him (the patient) with your back towards the North, and your feet close to his; you must place, without pressure, both your thumbs on the plexus of nerves of the epigastrium, and stretch your fingers towards the hypochondrium. It is beneficial occasionally to move your fingers on the sides, and especially in the regions of the spleen. After having continued this exercise for about a quarter of an hour you should change your mode of operating, according to the condition of your patient. For example, if it be a malady of the eyes, you place your left hand on the right temple of the sufferer, then present your thumbs to the open eyes of the patient and pass them down the nose and round the eyes. For violent headache, one thumb on the forehead, the other on the back of the head. So for all pains which are felt in other parts of the body, one hand always on one side, the other hand on the opposite side . . . ."

Controversy raged over Mesmer's methods of practice and he left Vienna for Paris where he arrived in 1778 and tried to convince the Royal Society of Medicine of the validity of his methods. Despite many reported cures dispute continued and a Commission was appointed by the Royal Society to look into Mesmer's claims and methods. Benjamin Franklin, who had arrived in France in 1778 on a mission to secure French military aid for George Washington, was a member of the Commission appointed by Louis XVI to report on the claims of "animal magnetism". The commission did not pronounce in favour of Mesmer and he left Paris in 1781, a disappointed man. The conclusions of the commission are of interest as they are relevant both to faith healing, hypnotism and psychotherapy as we see them practiced in our day.

"That which we have learned, or, at least, that which has been proved to us in a clear and satisfactory manner, by the examination of the process of Magnetism, is that man can act upon man at any time, and almost at will by striking his imagination; that the simplest gestures and signs can have the most powerful effects; and that the action of man upon the imagination may be reduced to an art, and conducted with method, upon subjects who have faith."

HERBAL REMEDIES

*"The rose distils a healing balm
The beating pulse of pain to calm."*
>   *Thomas Moore. Odes of Anacreon.
>   Ode 1v.*

Herbal remedies are the most delightful remedies known to man. Their use is almost as old as man himself. They call to mind the freshness of a garden in spring and the sweet scents of the summer air. Even if you have never taken any interest in herbal remedies there will be some herbs of which you are probably aware and one of these may well be chamomile. It is among the oldest favorites in garden herbs and has been grown for centuries. Revered in ancient times it reveals its presence when walked upon by the strong scent of apples. Its presence is thought to be beneficial to a garden and it used to be regarded as the "Plants Physician" since drooping plants were said to revive when a herb of chamomile was placed near them. Medicinally, chamomile tea is used for its gentle, soothing effect. It is particularly recommended for indigestion, colic and periodic headache to mention but a few of its reputed healing properties.

Nicholas Culpeper who died in 1654 was apprenticed to an apothecary and is remembered chiefly for his book "Herbal". He was very keen on the study of astrology and tells us under what planets the "simples" or single herbs used for medicinal purposes grow and of their good and bad qualities. He informs us that a "decoction of red roses with white wine . . . is very good for head-ache and pains in the eyes, ears, throat and gums." The idea of roses in the treatment of headache paints an appealing picture which in itself could give solace to the headache sufferer.

Pennyroyal is a species of mint which was recommended in Roman times as being more conducive to health than roses, and thought to be particularly efficacious in the treatment of headaches and giddiness.

Like roses, anenomes conjure up pleasing visions of garden plots, colour and sunlight. Tincture of anenome is recommended for the treatment of neuralgia and headache. Catmint, which should be infused but never boiled, is another herb which is used for the same symptoms.

Self heal is another herb which has been used for the treatment of headache. Culpeper explained the name "Self-heal" with the words "Self-Heal, whereby when you are hurt, you may heal yourself". Culpeper recommends that the juice of self-heal be "used with oil of roses to annoint the temples and forehead (and) is very effectual to remove the headache, and the same mixed with honey of roses cleaneth and healeth ulcers in the mouth and throat".

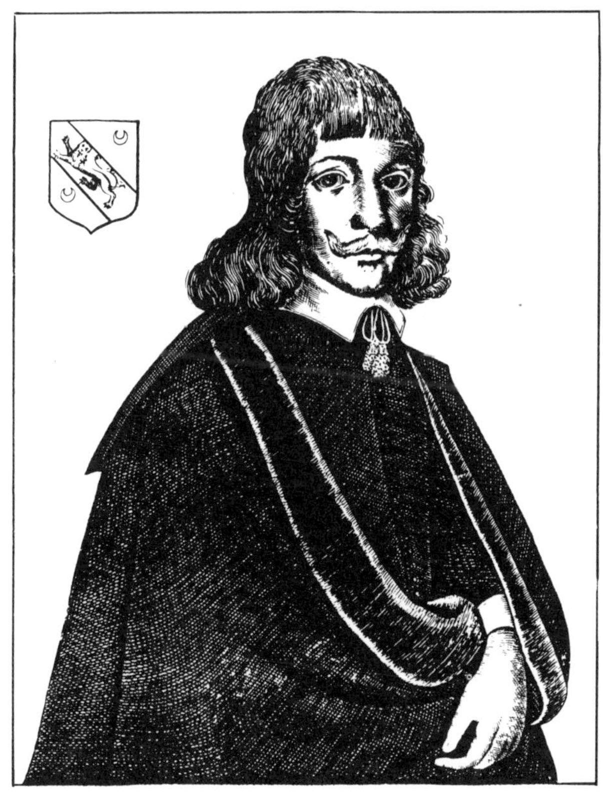

Nicholas Culpeper.

An infusion of the flowers of the herb Feverfew is said to allay sensitivity to pain and relieve faceache or earache. Feverfew received a great deal of publicity in Britain in the late nineteen seventies, when a doctor's wife in Wales reported that the severe attacks of migraine from which she had suffered for years were relieved after she had eaten up to three leaves of this common weed daily in a bread and butter sandwich, to which she added parsley to take away the bitter taste. Five months of this treatment were necessary before the lady noticed any improvement in her symptoms and during the same period of time she greatly reduced her intake of ergotamine tartrate. This reduction probably contributed in no small measure to the lessening of her headaches. Ergotamine compounds should be used warily and sparingly.

Ergot is obtained from the fungus Claviceps purpurea. Claviceps purpurea grows on a number of grasses. Ergot, however, is usually obtained from rye. Ergot contains a number of alkaloids of which the most important are ergonovine, ergotoscine and ergotamine.

In the past chronic poisoning with ergot occurred frequently in people fed on rye that was infected with the fungus. A village baker could be responsible for poisoning a whole community and the suffering must have been severe. Ergot poisoning was probably the cause of the great plague of Athens in the fifth century before Christ. The symptoms of ergot poisoning include burning and tingling in the hands and feet. For this reason it used to be called St. Anthony's fire. The name was derived from the Saint to whom supplications for relief were made. Ergot poisoning could result in peripheral gangrene with resultant gross deformity and loss of the extremities. The last known epidemic of ergotism was in 1816 but sporadic cases are still reported from time to time and can result from therapy with ergot compounds.

Ergot has a direct action on blood vessels and causes them to constrict. It is this constricting action of ergot which relieves the pain of migraine attacks. Unfortunately it can, on rare occasions and with protracted use, result in peripheral gangrene in the limbs.

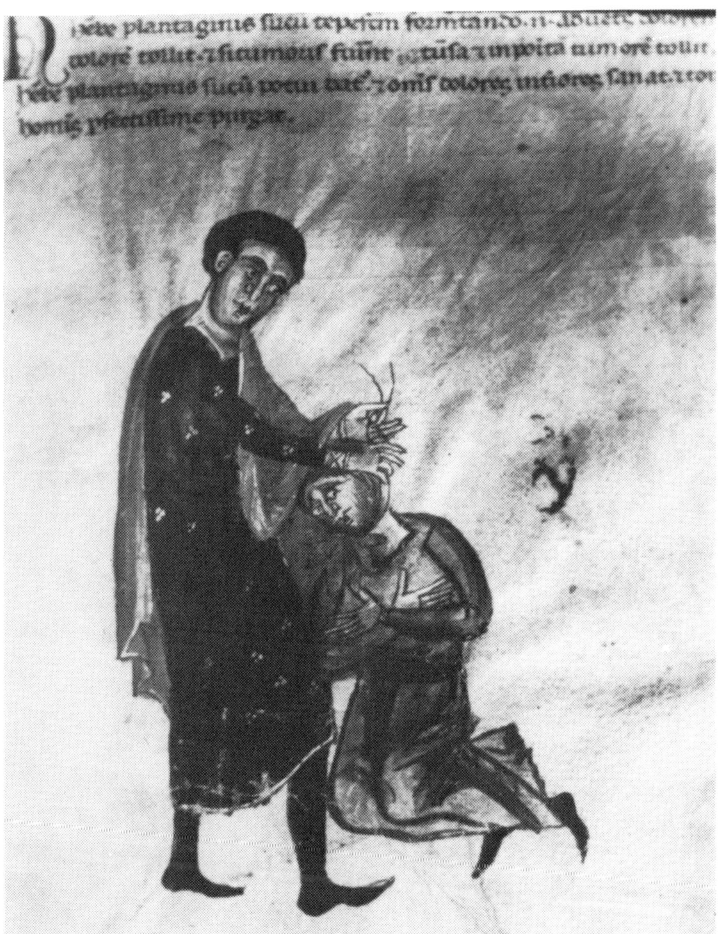

"Plaintain root, hung round the neck, takes away pain of the head marvelously"
13th Century

As one might, by now, have come to expect, Culpeper again, has a remedy for St. Anthony's fire. He reminds us of his astrological interests as he writes about the herb Alkanets — "It is an herb under the dominion of Venus, and indeed one of her darlings, though somewhat hard to come by. It helps old ulcers, hot inflammations, burnings by common fire and St. Anthony's fire . . ."

In 1596 Thomas Cogan wrote "Of all the garden herbs none is of greater virtue than Sage". This herb has many medicinal uses, including the relief of nervous headache, for which purpose its leaves are infused to make tea.

One of the delights in reading about herbs is the enchanting names by which they are described. Self-heal, for example, is also known as Heart of the Earth and Blue Curls. Among several other names the herb silver weed is also called Prince's Feathers and Trailing Tansy. It would seem fitting that we leave this short section on herbal remedies with thoughts of scarlet poppies in golden corn. For one of the synonyms by which the red poppy is known is Headache.

REFERENCES

1. Printed for J. Starkey, at the Miter in Fleet Street between the Middle Temple-Gate and Temple Bar 1666.

BIOFEEDBACK AND HEADACHE

A new type of therapy has recently aroused considerable interest. It is called Biofeedback. This is a method of treatment in which sufferers from certain disorders gradually learn to acquire some control over some of their bodily functions previously thought to be unresponsive to conscious influences. For example, we would not normally expect to have any conscious control over our heart rate or to alter the level of our blood pressure by mental concentration. The techniques of biofeedback consist of practical methods of achieving a state of mind over matter. The essence of biofeedback is, of course, psychological and the feedback consists of methods devised to inform the patient about how successful his or her efforts at control are proving to be. Thus an electromyograph which is an instrument designed to record muscle tension is used in some types of relaxation therapy which is used in tension headache. This provides a visual recording of muscular tension and the patient is able to note a decrease in this tension as his efforts in implementing the techniques used in biofeedback therapy take effect. A visual recording system could be used in a similar way to illustrate changes in pulse rate or blood pressure where therapy is being directed at achieving changes in them.

It does not take much imagination to realise that if one can link psychological factors with physical changes an individual could manipulate this ability to his or her advantage. Taking this to extremes one could cite the example of the elderly widow who has palpitations and goes deathly white every time her only son mentions his possible marriage. Consciously or unconsciously she has become a master in this art of mind over matter. Not surprisingly, the biofeedback method has particular application to psychosomatic disorders! These are disorders where mental states can influence the physical. While headache sufferers are no more neurotic than the rest of the population there is no doubt that the incidence of headache is often related to psychological factors. The most common type of headache is tension headache which results from a tightening of the muscles in the head and neck in response to tension or strain. Relaxation biofeedback therapy has produced encouraging results in tension headache. Various biofeedback techniques have been used in attempts to alleviate migraine. Probably the most commonly used method is one in which patients learn and practice hand warming techniques. An increasing ability to produce a rise in finger tip temperature is associated with a symptomatic improvement. A temperature monitor provides a visual recording of temperature changes and in this way the patient is able to see the results of efforts made and encouraged to maintain or improve them.

One could, of course, argue that biofeedback has certain similarities with meditation. In both one acquires a mastery over ones bodily reactions as well as over ones powers of concentration. While biofeedback techniques aim at controlling physical reactions it is obvious that a reduction in mental stress will also reduce these reactions and be likely to lead to a physical improvement. It is likely that meditation would produce equally successful results but the techniques of biofeedback provide a more tangible and generally applicable approach to this type of therapy.

REMARKS ON RESEARCH

"We travel not for trafficking alone;
By hotter winds our fiery hearts are fanned:
For lust of knowing what should not be known
We make the Golden Journey to Samarkand."
James Elroy Flecker (1884-1915).

Whenever it arises in general conversation the subject of medical research evokes immediate emotional reactions. Either "they" are not doing enough about "it", or "they" are always experimenting on you. It is not unusual to hear both criticisms levelled in almost the same breath. Interest is usually immediately focused on exciting areas of research such as heart transplant surgery. This interest soon abates, however. Fed as we are on a daily diet of death, violence and destruction we rapidly come to accept the most recent dramatic event whatever it may be. Within a short space of time we barely notice the small print in the paper which reports on the latest heart transplant survivor or the first test tube baby. But let us leave the emotional impact of medical research aside and consider the need for research.

Obviously it is necessary, you will say, because

without it our knowledge of disorders will stand still. Considering the atom bomb and atmospheric pollution as two of our current end products of advancing knowledge one might be forgiven for wondering whether the pursuit of knowledge is not without its drawbacks. But the same curiosity which has driven men forward to make these advances has also led to the steam engine, wireless waves, vaccination against smallpox and the prevention of rickets. We cannot decide in advance the direction in which man's curiosity should lead him and can only hope that good sense and sound judgement will enable new discoveries to be rightly used.

The search for knowledge is essential in our universities and other centers of learning. The undertaking of research implies inquiry and a constant seeking for the answers to questions. Unless teachers and students are encouraged to adopt this approach to problems, learning will rapidly become routine and stagnation will occur. For this reason research is undertaken in most university departments and the importance of a quest for knowledge for its own sake is recognized.

A classic example of this thirst for knowledge was Gregor Johann Mendel. Born in Austria in 1822 he entered the Augustinian monastery in Brunn at the age of twenty-one and was ordained as a priest five years later. He was partly a self-taught scientist but also studied at the University of Vienna from 1851 to 1853. He failed to pass the examination for a teacher's license but taught natural science in the technical high school for twelve years until in 1868 he was elected abbot of his monastery.

During the years when he was teaching at the technical school he was also carrying out patient meticulous research, crossing varieties of the garden pea in the monastery garden. He carefully noted the way in which differences in single characters such as tallness and shortness, seed shape and seed size were transmitted through succeeding generations of the pea plants. It is not difficult to imagine the endless patience and minute observation required to undertake this time consuming work. In 1856

Mendel published his experimental results and propounded the theory of inheritance which he had deduced from them. Acknowledgement of the major importance of his work which forms the basis of modern genetics, came only after his death. Mendel died in 1884 with his great scientific achievements unrecognized. Doubtless he found his earthly reward in the dedication of his labors to the glory of his Creator but his quiet perserverance and painstaking efforts remain an inspiration to us all.

Mendel may have had some inkling of the pratical application of the results of his resarch to the future of mankind, but certainly he was given no encouragement to make him think that this might be so. He carried out his work because he needed to know. He thirsted for knowledge.

Strong personal motives may drive a research worker forward but many other factors also play a role in the world of research. Chance is not the least of these. Even here, however, the chance occurrence has to be observed by the persistently curious mind or it will be overlooked. Had Alexander Fleming in 1928 tossed aside the culture plates on which no staphylococcal organisms had grown the world might not have reaped the benefits of penicillin. Eleven years after Fleming had first observed the curious mould which inhibited bacterial growth, penicillin was synthesized by Ernst Chain and Howard Florey. In 1945 the three men shared the Nobel Prize for medicine.

In 1890 a Dutch physician called Christiaan Eijkman was working in a military hospital in Java. He fed some domestic fowl on polished rice which was also the diet provided for his patients who were suffering from beri beri. The symptoms of beri beri resemble those of a multiple neuritis, affecting chiefly the lower limbs, with skin tenderness, muscle wasting and paralysis. The circulation becomes impaired and dropsy develops. The fowl in the hospital courtyard also developed weakness of the legs and head retraction. Then a new cook was appointed. He refused to supply military polished rice for the fowl and their diet was changed to whole grain civilian rice. Eijkman observed that they recovered from their symptoms. He became the first person to produce a dietary deficiency disease experimentally and to put forward the concept of "essential food factors", later called vitamins. He showed that there was something present in very small amounts in the germ and pericarp of rice that protected fowls from a disease resembling beri beri. This led to the discovery and eventual synthesis of thiamine. This is part of the Vitamin B complex and its absence in the diet leads to the symptoms of beri beri.

But let us return to the field of headache research. Here most of the effort has been concentrated on the problem of migraine. This is because the causes of migraine are so diverse, the mechanism of an attack so little understood and the effects of the disorder often so disabling.

Research into migraine is rather different from research into other disorders. Patients with migraine are rarely admitted to hospital for this complaint and are therefore seldom in the right place at the right time for the appropriate research techniques to be used. You can imagine, for example, how difficult it is to carry out blood flow studies during an acute attack of migraine with all the complicated equipment required at a specific momemt which cannot be arranged in advance. One neurologist tells the amusing tale of how a patient of his with frequent, severe migraine attacks volunteered to be admitted to hospital to take part in a research project. He became the proud reciopient of a magnificant pullover which she knitted him while she sat in the ward, day after day, waiting in vain for an attack to develop.

The problems of studying patients in migraine attacks has been partially solved by the setting up of migraine clinics for the treatment of patients in attacks. One of the first Headache Clinics began in Florence more than 30 years ago. Today, there are several clinics in the United States and in Britain and more have started in other parts of the world. In 1976, for example, migraine clinics were opened in Brussels and Amsterdam. These clinics are obviously the most suitable places in which to try new therapies for migraine and clinical trials are a routine part of their work. In addition, most clinics also follow their own particular lines of research.

There are a number of ways in which research into any disorder can be approached. The epidemiological approach has been commonly used in the study of headache. Epidemiology is the study of the incidence of a disease and the factors relating to its incidence. For example epidemiological studies pointed to the relationship between lung cancer and smoking.

A number of epidemiological studies have been carried out on the incidence of headache. These all confirm the fact that women suffer from headaches more than men and that the chief cause of headache is stress.

One has to remember that the findings in epidemiological surveys require careful interpretation and can be influenced by a large number of factors. This comment is illustrated by the recent findings of a survey in Finland in which the sauna bath was reported as the second most common cause of headache!

Research into migraine extends into every branch of medical science. Adequate financial support, the availability of the necessary techniques and skilled personnel are all essential to research. And in clinical research, particularly in the headache field, there is the constant difficulty of finding willing and suitable patient volunteers! Any or all of these factors will influence what can be achieved.

The greater part of research work consists of steady plodding with routine laboratory work and clinical observation. This, in itself, rarely leads to any major advances but it provides the foundations on which original ideas or hypotheses can be based. The essence of the scientific method is to prove or disprove these hypotheses by research. Whether or not absolute proof of anything is possible is, of course, the province of philosophy, but scientifically speaking, when a hypothesis has been proved or at least became generally accepted, the hypothesis becomes known as a theory. Possibly the words of Benjamin Franklin are appropriate to this train of thought "But in this world nothing can be said to be certain, except death and taxes".

HEADACHES IN HISTORY

Poets, philosophers, statesmen and kings — there have been headache sufferers among them all. It is fascinating to speculate on the way in which the effects of illness may have influenced the course of human history. George III provides us with an example of this. Eight years after his army had been defeated in the battle at Yorktown, and America had secured her independence, he had an attack of what his family and his people considered to be insanity. During the latter part of his life he suffered recurrent breakdowns and in 1810 the Prince of Wales was appointed Regent. Eventually George became totally blind and very deaf and is said to have spent his time wandering about his rooms in a purple dressing gown. We now believe that he was suffering from porphyria but in his day there was no means of recognizing this rare disorder.

Alexander the Great is thought to have suffered from migraine. This did not prevent him from having a major effect on the course of world history. Alexander was taught by Aristotle, and ascended the throne of Greece at the age of 20 following his father's assasination. During his brief life from 356 B.C. to 323 B.C. his conquests enabled him to spread the language and civilization of Greece throughout the ancient world.

We can only speculate about the health of Henry VIII. It is likely that the ravages of syphilis, which was rampant in his day, were responsible for the physical and mental changes which gradually transformed him from a charming, athletic, intelligent and artistic young man into an evil-tempered, corpulent tyrant. Soon after his second wife Anne Boleyn gave birth, in 1533, to a daughter, later to become the first Queen Elizabeth, Henry developed an intractable ulcer on his thigh. At the same time he is reported to have suffered from intense headaches and these combined with the pain of his ulcer can have done little to improve either his temper or his judgement. The daughter of his first marriage to Catherine of Aragon was Mary Tudor, later named "Bloody Mary", an account of the persecutions carried out during her three year reign. The name might equally well have described the many misfortunes which dogged the life of this unhappy woman from the cradle to the grave. One of these misfortunes was the fact that she was never well and that her activities were marred by the very severe headaches that afflicted her.

Three hundred years later Queen Victoria and her daughter provided us with incidental accounts of their headaches in correspondence which makes fascinating reading. The strains and stresses of their lives were manifold. As far as the Crown Princess of Prussia was concerned the stifling atmosphere of the royal palaces was undoubtedly one of them. On January 1st, 1869 she wrote to her mother "The heat of rooms in the palaces and the smells and want of ventilation turns me quite sick" and on April 17th of the same year ". . . the soiree was so stiflingly hot and so late that I had a violent headache all day yesterday". A year earlier she had written to her mother "I do hope your visit to London will go off well and that the heat and the unwonted exertion will not be too much for you and give you one of your bad headaches. I am indeed distressed to hear that the blood so easily gets to your head and that your feet swell." Swollen feet and headaches present the

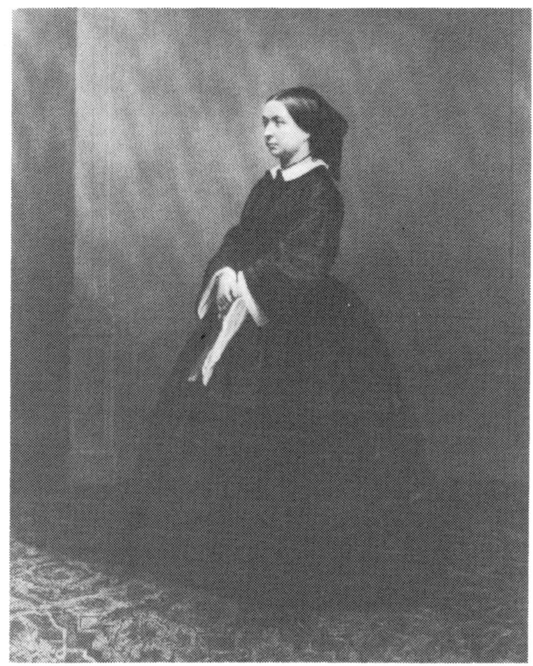

Queen Victoria. 1819-1901.

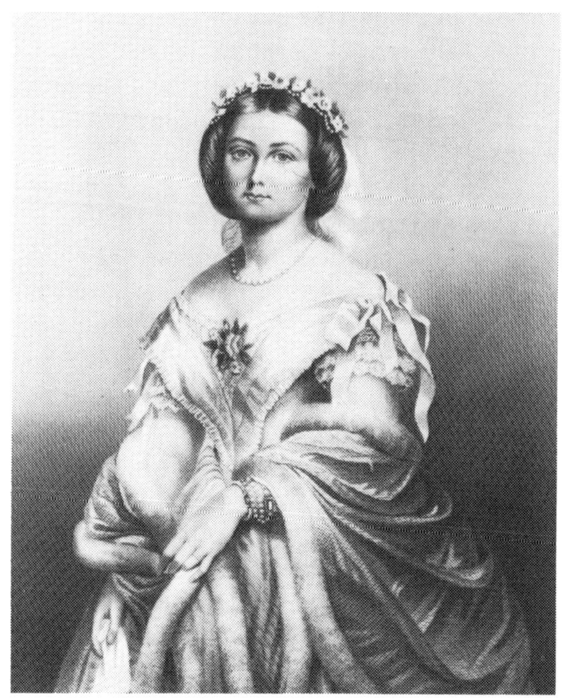

Crown Princess of Prussia. 1840-1901.

Queen in rather a prosaic light but she herself was equally down to earth in her comments to her daughter in the same year when she wrote of her ever increasing family "the seventh grand-daughter and fourteenth grandchild becomes a very uninteresting thing — for it seems to me to go on like the rabbits in Windsor Park"!

It is hard to tell whether Queen Victoria and her daughter suffered from migraine, which is often familial or from tension headache. The nausea so often referred to in association with their headaches suggests a diagnosis of migraine. In 1867, for example, Queen Victoria wrote "Yesterday morning after breakfast (with a very bad headache, which lasted all day as it had done the day before, and disgust for food) I took a drive round the grounds . . ."[1]

In 1801 Thomas Jefferson became the third President of the United States. He began his career by being admitted to the bar in 1767 but turned to politics two years later. He claimed to be the author of the declaration of independence which was signed on July 4th 1776. Jefferson died fifty years later on the day of the month that he had made historic, July 4th. He is of particular interest to us in the light of some words that he wrote to a friend which suggest that he suffered severely from migraine since he refers to

"An attack of the periodical headache which came on me about a week ago rendering me unable as yet either to write or read without great pain."

It used to be thought that migraine sufferers were particularly intelligent. This is untrue. The commonly held but erroneous belief arose from the fact that the more intelligent migraine sufferers are more articulate and thus a number of famous astronomers and scientists have left us accounts of their attacks. These have related largely to the weird and often visual prodromal symptoms preceding the headache phase of an attack. During these prodromal symptoms of classical migraine some patients feel themselves to be changing in size. Lewis Carroll suffered from migraine and may have been describing his own prodromal symptoms when he tells us about Alice feeling as though she was shutting up like a telescope after she had fallen down the rabbit hole and drank the bottle labelled "Drink me" and opening out again when she ate the small cake beautifully marked in currants with the words "Eat me'.

Philosophical thoughts have not spared some of our greatest thinkers from headaches. It is said that every book written by Friederich Nietzsche, the German philosopher who lived from 1844 to 1900, represented a triumph over his headaches. In the light of this personal suffering it is perhaps surprising that he proclaimed that only the strong should survive and that human sympathy perpetuates the unfit and mediocre. A century later Simone Weil, a French philosophical writer with a deep mystical feeling for the Catholic faith pondered on organized religion. Like her father, she, too, suffered from migraine and her recurrent bouts of severe pain interfered with her teaching of philosophy. She described her suffering as a "pain situated around the central point of the nervous system, at the point of junction between soul and body, which goes on even through sleep, never ceasing for a second."

Headache sufferers sometimes complain that the glare of bright sunlight or snow increases the intensity of their symptoms. Edward Wilson would have known about this. He combined his skills as a physician, naturalist and explorer when he went to the Antartic with Scott in the "Discovery" in 1901. Nine years later he returned there. He perished with Scott and his companions on their return journey from the Pole in 1912. There are references to Edward Wilson's symptoms in the chronicles of that ill-fated journey.

Volumes could be written on the headaches of famous men and women. They would include Peter the Great, Blaise Pascal, and Rudyard Kipling among countless others. Despite their headaches many of them rose to great heights and triumphed over adversity. Perhaps the words of Nietzsche who himself suffered so acutely are appropriate "What does not destroy me, makes me stronger".

---

[1]from the private corresplondence of Queen Victoria and the Crown Princess of Prussia (1865-1871). Edited by Rober Fulford. London. Evan Brothers Limited.

SUMMING UP

Long, long ago, when I was a child, I heard someone say that three of the saddest words in the English language are "I had hoped". The words are still in my mind. I had hoped that the end of my book would consist of a grand summing up containing profound thoughts on the subject of headache. These profound thoughts (or the lack of them) have circled around my brain until they have given me a headache. For if you have read through the book you will know that tension is the most common cause of headaches.

Now, sadder but probably wiser, I am forced to admit that I cannot express myself better than the much quoted Robin and Sparrow:

'Said the Robin to the Sparrow
"I would really like to know why these anxious
    human beings
Rush around and worry so."
Said the Sparrow to the Robin
"I think that it must be
That they have no heavenly Father
Such as cares for you and me!" '

If, like the Robin and Sparrow we know that we have a heavenly Father, what difference does it make?

It will certainly not make our problems disappear. Disappointments, failures and heartaches will still be with us. But our attitude will change and we may gradually learn to view things more in the light of eternity. It will make us feel less competitive to our neighbors and more tolerant to them, as children of the same Father. Thus the tension in our lives will lessen. For what the world needs most of all is more love — real love which helps us to apply ourselves to seeking the well being of others. And if the injustices and inequalities which are so apparent in life threaten to overwhelm us, then while doing what we can to amend them we can remember that:

"Though the mills of God grind slowly,
   yet they grind exceedingly small;
Though with patience he stands waiting with
   exactness grinds He all."

Friedrich Von Logau (1605-1655)

Sinngedichte 111. ii
(translated H.W. Longfellow)